Pra...
How to Sur...
Step-by-...

This book was so compelling that I had to put it down. Frequently. Starting early on, I stopped reading and went to work with what I had learned. First, to assemble essential information from several sources about myself — I live most of the time alone — in case I needed emergency help. It took an hour, and made me feel safer. I came back to learn more from later sections (tip: use the speaker button on your phone when you call 911). I wished the extensive practical advice for caregivers had been given to me on the day my wife was diagnosed with dementia. One sentence near the end of the book, about surviving natural disasters, made me laugh out loud. The authors wrote, "Do this right now, before reading further." They didn't have to tell me. But no joke: this book could save your life.

– *Gurney Williams III,*
Journalist and Public Speaker
Advocate for the Alzheimer's Association

Many have not thought of these critical steps and necessities until a disaster is on their doorstep. This incredible book benefits both civilians and emergency service workers. There's more in this book than even many responders know!

– *Alexander Nicholas*
Assistant Fire Chief

As a psychotherapist/hypnotherapist who also works in a hospital O.R. with surgical patients before and during surgery, I welcome this book. I have seen patients suffering from delayed procedures because of a lack of immediately available information and documents, which should have been on hand when they arrived at the hospital.

This clearly written, informational book covers what you need to know to be prepared and able to respond quickly and efficiently to an emergency. It's so basic and needed, it's hard to believe that we didn't have it all along. No one should be without it!

– *Alexandra Chalif, MS, MP*
Psychotherapy/Hypnotherapy/NLP
Medical Hypnosis in Surgery

A Family Caregiver's Guide

How to
Survive
911
Medical Emergencies

Step-by-Step Before, During, and After!

Nancy May
Robert Antonion

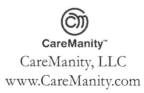

CareManity, LLC
www.CareManity.com

Disclaimer: All rights reserved. No part of this book may be reproduced by any mechanical, photographic, or electronic process, or in the form of a photographic recording; nor may it be stored in a retrieval system, transmitted, or otherwise copied for public or private use — other than for "fair use" as brief quotations embodied in articles and reviews — without prior written permission of the publisher CareManity, LLC, and the authors.

Notice of Liability: The intent of the authors is only to offer information of a general nature to help you, the reader, in your quest for emotional, physical, and spiritual well-being. In the event you or anyone else uses any of the information in this book for yourself, a family member, friend, or other person, the authors and publisher assume no responsibility for any actions taken by any readers or users of this book.

This book is intended to serve as a general guide for caregivers to better prepare, address, and follow up before, during, and after making a 911 call. It is not intended to replace professional medical, legal, or financial advice. This guide is not intended as a way to provide diagnosis or treatment, nor does it dispense medical advice or prescriptive use of any techniques as a form of treatment for physical, emotional, or medical problems, either directly or indirectly. Always seek the advice and guidance of medical, legal, and financial professionals and advisors as well as that of your family members in any emergency, life-care, or medical situation.

The information in this book is distributed on an "as is" basis, without warranty. There are no guarantees that you will have success with the ideas expressed in this book. While every precaution has been taken in the preparation of this book, neither the authors nor CareManity LLC, shall have any liability to any person or entity with respect to any liability, loss, or damage caused or alleged to be caused directly or indirectly by the information or websites contained in this book.

Trademarks: Throughout this book, trademarked names are used. Rather than put a trademark symbol in every occurrence of a trademarked name, we are using the names only in an editorial fashion and to the benefit of the trademark owner, with no intention of infringement of the trademark. Where those designations appear in this book, the designations have been printed in initial caps.

© Copyright 2020, CareManity, LLC, all rights reserved.
Published in the United States by CareManity, LLC
For more information about CareManity, LLC, please visit our website at www.caremanity.com

Library of Congress Cataloging-in-Publication Data is available on file.
ISBN: 978-1-7348416-0-2

The future depends on what you do today.

—*Mahatma Gandhi*

Contents

Acknowledgements	3
Introduction	4
How to Use This Guide	8
Part 1: Prepare to Get Help	**11 – 32**
Prepare Everyone: The File of Life	12
Prepare Everyone: The Go Bag	16
Prepare Your Home	23
Prepare Your Environment	28
Part 2: Prepare to Give Help	**33 – 46**
Learn Basic First Aid	35
Household First Aid Kits	38
Learn How to Do CPR and Use an AED	43
Part 3: Getting Help	**47 – 70**
Getting Help From 911	48
Helping Out	54
What to Do Before the Ambulance Leaves	57
At the Hospital Emergency Department	61
Special Considerations for Elderly Patients	65
A Note About Hospital-Induced Delirium	67
Part 4: What's Next	**71 – 90**
For Your Charge	72
Getting Discharged From the Hospital	73
Discharge to Home	75
Discharge to a Care Facility	78
What's Next for You	85
Part 5: Getting Help in a Time of Disaster	**91 – 105**
Final Note	106
Special Thanks and About the Authors	107
Reader Notes	**108 – 111**

Nobody ever wishes
they had prepared less for an emergency.

—*Anonymous*

Acknowledgements

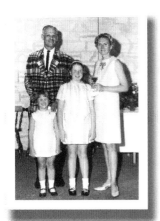

This book is dedicated to the memory of my dad, Stuart, who passed away at age 99, and to my mom, Audrey, who, thankfully, is still with us at the time of this publishing. I hope she will be with us for many more years to come.

Through 12-plus years of being a long-distance caregiver, my family has been supported by and witnessed the dedication of numerous 911 emergency responders. They, along with other medical professionals, inspired us to write this guide book. It is intended to help those of you who provide continuing care for elderly, frail, ill, or infirm family members, loved ones, friends, and neighbors, as well as those who do so as a paid or voluntary service.

A special thank you goes out to my incredible homecare aides and long-distance right hands who've helped me through these years: Millie, Addie, Iris, Kayla, Nurse Sarah, Pete, and Aiden. My thanks, of course, go out to all my family members, friends, colleagues, professional and medical advisors, and acquaintances who've been there, giving me support, advice, and patience through stressful times.

We at CareManity, LLC, also want to thank those who made this guide for family caregivers possible.

Nancy May
Nancy May
CEO, Co-Founder
CareManity, LLC

Introduction

Now, after 50 years, almost everyone in the United States has access to the 911 system. Since its inception, it has evolved into a well-coordinated, highly structured emergency response system, utilizing trained personnel who can quickly receive, categorize, and prioritize calls from those in need, and promptly dispatch help. Even if we just talk about medical emergencies, countless people owe their lives to the 911 system. Yet countless others never made it through, despite calling or having someone else call 911 for them.

Why? Some succumbed because of the emergency situation they were already in: things had already occurred that could not be fixed, or got worse before help arrived, or got worse after help arrived. For many others, either they or those who tried to get help for them were unprepared or lacked the knowledge to "clear the way" for responders to get them care timely.

The odds of surviving, for many, could have been improved if they, or those caring for them, had made preparations in advance, had an understanding of what to expect along the way and what could go wrong, and acquired the skills needed to help out before, during, and after help arrived.

Calling 911 in an emergency may be the most important thing you ever do. However, it is only one tool to get you and your charge through a medical emergency. Also, relying solely on 911 in an emergency, or using it incorrectly to get help, may not turn out as well as you might hope or expect.

This guide lays out a smarter *process* to improve the odds that you and your charge(s) have successful outcomes (i.e., survive) when going through a medical emergency. This process requires you and yours to prepare to survive. That means getting yourself, your family, your charges, your home, and your environment ready for a medical emergency. You need to make your home and environment "responder ready." You need to learn how to give critical aid that keeps your charge stable until professional help arrives. You need to know how to get responders to your charge quickly and be as helpful to them as you can while they are there. It's also important to know how to get prompt care at — and "work" — a hospital emergency department. Finally, you need to plan for and get through the recovery process with your charge and take care of yourself, too. That includes learning from the experience so you can improve what you know and better handle things the next time. It also includes assessing the emergency's impact on you, the caregiver, so that you can successfully recover yourself.

The Process: Prepare to Get Help

Prepare everyone you care for by getting together the information and items you will need for yourself and your charges when a medical emergency happens.

Getting the materials together is not difficult, but it can take time to gather everything. If it seems too overwhelming to do everything at once, do what needs to be done bit by bit, focusing on progress. Budget time to get organized and prepared, but be steady about it. Medical emergencies will not wait for your schedule. Visualize that a clock is always ticking and that the odds will not get better unless you are prepared.

You will need to set up **File of Life** packets for each person living full time in the household. That will require going through documentation; interviewing your charges, if possible; getting it all written down correctly; and placing those files where they can be found and used easily.

You will need to set up a **Go Bag** that has important information, documents, and other items that hospital staff and your charge will need to get the right care promptly. This will require going through even more documentation, making copies, and putting them into folders, binders, or whatever works to keep them organized and up-to-date. You may also want to decide, with your charge(s), what items to take along that will give them comfort and help lower their stress.

Every household should also have an organized, up-to-date **First Aid Kit** on hand. A handy, well-thought-out First Aid Kit can help keep a minor mishap from becoming a medical emergency or a serious injury from becoming life-threatening.

In the following pages, we've laid out what many of these things are, why you need them, and how to put them together so they are ready to use. These items, the information you'll find here, and the courses that we recommend should be thought of as **life-saving tools**.

Prepare Your Home and Environment

Do a walk-through of your home for obstacles and impediments that may prevent responders from getting to your charge promptly. Get out and meet with responders and all those whom you think may be able to help you and yours later on. Find out what relevant emergency resources are available in your neighborhood, community, town, county, or city.

Prepare to Give Help

Improving the odds for a good outcome means not waiting for help to arrive before doing something yourself that could save a life. Learn the skills that can keep someone alive, or at least stable, until responders get there. In an emergency, time is critical to survival.

Developing these skills, at the minimum, require knowing how to administer **Basic First Aid and Cardiopulmonary Resuscitation**.

Know How to Get Help

Know **the way 911 works** and what responders will need from you when they arrive. Know what you need to do to help them do their jobs well. Understand **how emergency departments and hospital medical staff operate** and what they will need from you. This information is critical for getting faster attention and more precise treatment for your charge

Recovery and Learning

To complete the process, you need to learn how both your charge and you, the caregiver, can best recover from the emergency. Understand which changes, if any, need to be made in your charge's care, and adapt accordingly. Learn from the experience and make note of what you can do better next time. Finally, self-assess or get assistance in learning **what effects the emergency had on you**. Take those steps that work best for you to reduce stress and make you stronger and a better caregiver.

How to Use This Guide

This guide has been written for family caregivers like you to help you and yours improve the odds of getting a good outcome in an emergency (i.e., surviving). It is based on the experiences and knowledge of caregivers who've been through 911 emergencies, as well as that of first responders, emergency department doctors, nurses, and other health care professionals. To get the most from this book, *read, learn,* and then *take action*.

First, **read** everything in these pages and **learn** what to do before, during, and after an emergency. Once you become familiar with this guide's key points, **take action**: decide which of the actions recommended in these pages you can begin to do now. Some can be done easily, while others may take more time and commitment. The more you do, the better prepared you will be and the better off everyone may be later on. As you complete tasks, mark off the check boxes provided alongside items and suggestions listed throughout this book.

Getting everything prepared and ready for any emergency will raise your **confidence**, which will help you remain **calm** and in **control** when you need it most. Your confidence, in turn, will help those around you stay calm and be more helpful to you when you need them most.

Highlight ideas and specific page sections as you need to, and jot down notes in the blank pages at the end of this guide. However, be sure to put everything into practice that applies to you. Mark a date in your calendar every month to review and practice some of these tips. If you find yourself time-stretched, at least **review the summary pages in each section** and refresh what you've learned. Turn these tips into skills, and make those skills second nature.

As an **intelligent family caregiver**, you can play a critical role in improving the odds that the 911 emergency call you make turns out well for all involved. Begin the process of preparing by fighting through denial. It's important to admit to yourself that a medical emergency will probably happen, and not when you expect it. You hope that it won't, but you should assume that it will. With that in mind, start to do something. Prepare for a medical emergency now. It will make your life as a caregiver easier later and give you more time to focus on your charge's urgent care when it's needed most.

Finally, keep this guide in an easy-to-find place, such as in a kitchen drawer or on a bookshelf.

1

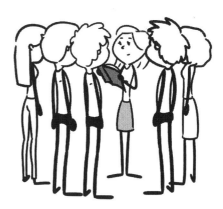

Prepare To Get Help

Prepare Everyone!

The File of Life: What Is It?
A **File of Life** is a card or sheet of paper that contains your charge's important medical information. It's best kept in some small, usually red (the universal emergency color) holder placed somewhere visible, where anyone can easily get to it, such as on the front or side of the home's refrigerator.

Why Have One?
Emergency responders will, most likely, immediately ask for this upon arriving at your home. They are also trained to look for one in an obvious place, usually on the home's refrigerator. Hospital emergency department personnel will also ask for this. It gives them quick, important background information to use to decide on how best to help you. It can save a lot of precious time in getting treatment to you wherever you are, or in getting you faster attention and care in the hospital. All medical professionals we've spoken with agree that having a **current File of Life could make a big difference in saving a life**. It's a good idea to get or make at least five copies of this for everyone living in the household.

How to Make (or Get) One
You can purchase a File of Life template online. Sometimes police, fire, or rescue departments have these available and supply them free of charge for local residents. You can also make your own File of Life by putting all the information (see below) on 3 x 5-inch cards, placing them in a clear plastic sandwich bag, and then putting them on your refrigerator door or side using a magnet, sticky hook, or even duct tape.

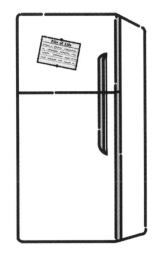

There are different File of Life templates out there. At a minimum, the file should include: **the person's name, date of birth, important medical conditions, allergies, a photo ID, and important phone numbers**. Below is a suggested checklist if you are just starting with a blank sheet of paper.

Clearly, and in large print, write down:

- ❑ Name (both legal and familiar)
- ❑ Gender
- ❑ Date of birth
- ❑ Home address
- ❑ Emergency contact names and phone numbers
- ❑ Social Security number
- ❑ Blood pressure average (high/medium/low)
- ❑ Medical ID bracelet (if there is one)
- ❑ All prescription drugs and dosage times — include all vitamins, supplements, and homeopathic and alternative remedies being used
- ❑ Medical summary: disease/afflictions/disabilities, recent significant changes, surgeries, and dates of each
- ❑ List of doctors, specialists, preferred hospital, emergency family contacts, aides, and their phone numbers
- ❑ Allergies/sensitivities to medications and equipment, such as latex gloves, alcohol, x-ray dye, foods, animals (like bees), and plants
- ❑ Implants, including: pacemakers, medical ports, stents, joints, prosthetic arms/legs, dental (loose teeth), etc. (include manufacturers, types, exact body locations, and dates)

- ❏ Notes on who has the Durable Power of Attorney (POA), medical directives, Do Not Resuscitate/Do Not Intubate orders (DNR/DNI*), Physician's Order for Life-Sustaining Treatment (POLST), legal guardianship, etc.
- ❏ Mental situation: dementia, Alzheimer's, autism, etc.
- ❏ Impairments, including use of glasses and hearing aids and mobility issues needing prosthetics, wheelchair, walkers, crutches, catheters, oxygen, or other mobility or life-supporting devices
- ❏ Medical insurance information and policy numbers

Always update all file packets every time there are any changes.

Many Emergency Medical Technicians (EMTs) will only accept an original or notarized copy of a DNR/DNI. Without this, they will begin resuscitation, whether you want it or not.

When to Use It

You should give a File of Life to responders immediately upon their arrival so that they can quickly understand the important medical conditions of the person in need. Keep two extra copies in your Go Bag, in case you need to give one to the emergency department doctors when you arrive there. The extras are just in case any get lost along the way. Keep at least one backup copy somewhere separately in the house.

It's also a good idea to take a File of Life (just the card or paper, not the holder) with you, **wherever you go**. Emergencies can happen anywhere, any time. Keep it in a wallet, purse, cell phone holder, car glove compartment, or inside whatever a person always takes with them. You can wrap it in plastic to prevent/reduce wear and damage. *That's right, five copies in total — for each member in the household!*

You can also download medical information apps for your cell phone, or take a photo of the File of Life and put it in an emergency file on your phone. Don't forget to update these when anything changes.

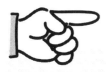

File of Life Summary

- A File of Life packet should contain a photo ID copy, name, address, gender, date of birth, medications used, allergies, doctors and family phone numbers, mental and physical disabilities, implants, power of attorney contact information, the location of medical directives, and insurance information.*

- Make File of Life packets (minimum of five) for each person living full time in your household. **Update each person's File of Life package** whenever there are any changes to medical, legal, or insurance information, or emergency contacts.

- Put one File of Life on the refrigerator or in an easy-to-reach location. Add the Go Bag location and responders' (direct dial/non-911) non-emergency numbers inside, or next to, the File of Life packet.

- In an emergency, give the person's File of Life to the responders as soon as they arrive.

- Put two of the five File of Life packets that you've made into each person's Go Bag. You can give one to the attending doctors in the emergency department when you arrive at the hospital.

- Keep one File of Life or equivalent with your charge wherever they go. Update all File of Life forms whenever there are any changes in the person's medical, legal, insurance, or financial status.

* *EMTs may require an original or notarized copy of your DNR, DNI, POLST. Keep copies with the File of Life or in the Go Bag.*

The Go Bag

What Is It?
A **Go Bag** is something in which you keep **important, detailed medical, legal, and insurance information**. If you think something may be helpful with your charge's care in the hospital, such as small personal and comfort items, include them in a separate bag together with your charge's Go Bag. Keep and carry all your detailed information in a large enough, easy-to-carry tote-like bag, large purse, or zippered folder

Why Have One?
Your Go Bag is similar to, but should not be confused with, a hospital bag typically advertised or referred to for expectant mothers. The Go Bag referred to in these pages should contain critical medical and legal information as well as documents to support medical staff questions in an emergency. It's not intended to support a patient's comfort for a long-term hospital stay.

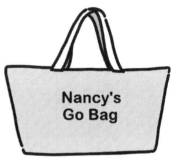

You need to store and safely carry this information (more than what is on a File of Life) with you, or with someone you trust, to the hospital's emergency department. This includes legal documents, insurance information, medical directives, medical histories (don't count on the hospital having any of your records), notes, results and information about past doctors' visits, assessments, lab test results, surgeries, implant information, etc.

Having all this important detailed information organized and with you in your Go Bag can help medical professionals give you and your charge prompt attention and appropriate care during and after a medical emergency. Doctors and emergency department personnel have told us that not having enough detailed information about your charge's current and past medical condition(s) and medications can significantly delay any help you may get in the emergency department. In addition, without this information, your chances of **getting the right treatment** may be lower, as medical staff may have to guess what's wrong and may have to provide unnecessary, time-consuming, and difficult exploratory tests.

If your charge has a cognitive impairment such as dementia or Alzheimer's disease, or does not manage stress well, bring small comfort and personal items with you to help reduce stress, anxiety, and even delirium in your charge while in the hospital.

How to Make (or Get) One

Since a Go Bag is meant to carry items for the needs of a specific person, it may be difficult to find a Go Bag that will remain suitable over time. You may need a larger or smaller one as time goes by. Don't concern yourself with making it perfect or fashionable.

When you put your Go Bag together, start by first gathering everything in one place, including the information and items you think you'll need to have (see the checklist below). Based on what you've laid out, you can figure out what size bag or tote you will need. It should be large enough to neatly carry all the items that you've decided need to be in there, with room for expansion.

Your Go Bag should be sturdy, so it doesn't break with repeated use. Label or tag each bag with the person's name.

Your Go Bag should include detailed medical, personal, legal, and insurance information. You'll need to decide, based on the type of document, whether you need an original, a notarized copy, or simply a photocopy. In most cases, a responder/EMT will need an original copy of a DNR/DNI for them not to perform CPR or to intubate your charge. Other documents include: their durable or basic POA, POLST, personal medical directive, or living will.

Here's a checklist of what your Go Bag should include:

○ **File of Life** — two copies (minimum) for the individual
○ Blank notebook, pens, and permanent marker (black or blue)
○ Binder, file folder, or large envelope that contains more detailed medical information, including:

- ❑ All prescription drugs and dosage times, including vitamins, supplements, and homeopathic and alternative remedies taken (if possible, include a list of medications that were previously prescribed, including dosage)
- ❑ List of doctors, specialists, aides, etc. and their addresses, and phone numbers
- ❑ Primary contacts (POA holder, guardians, primary family members), including other support people such as religious advisors and legal counsel
- ❑ Pharmacy information (backup prescriptions if lost)
- ❑ Medical history — diseases, afflictions, disabilities; recent significant changes; surgeries; and dates of occurrences (or estimates if you don't have exact dates)
- ❑ Normal vitals: high and low blood pressure, heart rate, oxygen levels
- ❑ Dates of doctors' visits and recommendations
- ❑ Most recent lab test results, including blood tests, x-rays, MRIs, etc.
- ❑ Allergies/sensitivities to medications or equipment (like latex gloves, alcohol wipes, powders, etc.)
- ❑ List of implants/devices used, including joints, stents, pacemakers, dental, infusion pumps, etc. (including their brands, serial numbers, body locations, and date placed)
- ❑ Mental situations — depression, anxiety, psychoses, dementia, Alzheimer's, etc.

- ☐ Mobility issues — for example, can/can't walk on their own, need stability assistance, need prosthetics, walkers, crutches, oxygen, catheters, etc.
- ☐ Impairments, including use of glasses or hearing aids

Legal Documents

- ☐ Complete copies of POA, durable POA, POLST, medical directives, DNR (original or notarized copy), DNI (original or notarized copy), living wills, legal guardianship, and other related documents.
- ☐ Social Security number
- ☐ Lawyer(s), names and phone number(s)
- ☐ Military service records (copies)
- ☐ Marriage certificates, verified copies, if possible

Financial/Insurance Documents

- ☐ Insurance cards, Medicare, Medicaid, supplemental insurance cards (copies)
- ☐ Funeral arrangements, funeral home contact numbers (if already made and purchased)

Information on Support People

- ☐ Neighbors and friends names, phone numbers, and email addresses
- ☐ Babysitter and dog/pet walker or sitter names, phone numbers and email addresses
- ☐ Transportation support: names and phone numbers

Other Items

You can include **small comfort and personal care items** and familiar keepsakes to help keep your charge relaxed and happy. If you anticipate needing such items, make sure you use a large enough bag or have a second bag strictly for those items. Keep them loosely fastened together so you don't forget to take both, or take the wrong one. These items may include:

- ❑ Prosthetics, glasses, hearing aids, urinary catheters, colostomy equipment, walkers, gait belts, compression socks, special shoes, etc.
- ❑ Particular hygiene items (dental, sanitary, etc.)
- ❑ Calming and mental support items: small plush toys for anxiety, pillow or blanket, cherished family photos
- ❑ Extra warming items (socks/booties/slippers)
- ❑ Cell phone (for your charge to use), device chargers, ear buds or small speaker, small blank notebook, pens

Keep these personally labeled bags (one for each household member) in a safe, but easily accessible, place, close to where you enter and exit the home.

Backup E-Copies

Most information that you would place in a Go Bag can also be copied into a cell phone by taking photos of each document and storing them in a photo folder. Scanning all documents and converting them to PDF format and emailing or texting them to the phone can also be effective. It's important to note that when/where originals are required, you will still need your physical Go Bag along with appropriate original information and/or specific details about your charge.

When Traveling

Take the Go Bag with you and your charge! If that's not practical:

- ❑ Make up a smaller, lighter **Traveling Go Bag** with all the same important information (and one File of Life).

❏ Forego comfort and personal items for portability.

❏ At the least, keep the File of Life with your charge whenever he/she travels anywhere.

When to Use It

Go Bags are meant to be a **portable source of vital information**. Go Bags should contain medical histories and more detail on conditions, procedures, diagnoses, assessments, disabilities, medical equipment needs, and so forth. When you need proof of who has guardianship, who has durable POA, or what your charge's medical wishes are, they should be in your Go Bag.

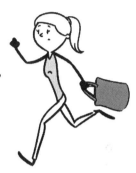

Always keep your Go Bag with you while in the hospital. This way you can quickly **pull out information you need** when asked for it by hospital doctors and/or administrators.

Emergency departments and hospitals can't be relied upon to have or gain access to your up-to-date information. Having all this in your Go Bag makes it easier for medical staff to make quicker, more accurate assessments and treatment plans. Having insurance information on hand can help you ask about coverage for different procedures and alternatives.

Comfort and personal items can go a long way in lowering fear, anxiety, and stress (your charge's and yours).

It's a good idea to take a Go Bag with you **whenever you go to any medical appointment**. Doctors don't always remember everything about you, or write everything down. Don't rely on your memory for when things happened in the past, what you were told, or what instructions you were given. You can more easily update Go Bag information right then.

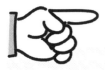

Go Bag Summary

- A **Go Bag** should be a sturdy tote, zipped folder, or a carryall that can contain detailed medical, legal, and financial information needed by the emergency department and hospital to provide treatment.

- **Two File of Life packets** should be kept there.

- A Go Bag should be **clearly labeled** or **tagged** for the person to whom it belongs.

- Place Go Bags where you can **quickly grab and take the right one(s) with you**.

- **Update all information** after any medical, legal, or financial changes occur.

- Go Bag information should be **backed up or photocopied and stored somewhere that's secure** and **separate** from each Go Bag.

- Go Bags can be used to **carry personal or comfort items** to keep a patient calmer or more comfortable while undergoing treatment.

- You can **make PDFs** or **take photos of all Go Bag information** and put them on your **cell phone**, but you **may still need originals** or **notarized copies**.

- For **travelers: take the Go Bag with you**. If impractical, make up a smaller information-only Go Bag to use when traveling. At the least, **keep the File of Life with your charge wherever you go**.

Prepare Your Home

The second part in preparing for a medical emergency is to make sure that responders can easily and reliably find you and get to your charge quickly. If a responder (fire, police, EMT) can't find where you are, they may be delayed or never get to you. If they can't get equipment to your charge easily, they may need to wait for backup such as more EMTs, police officers, or fire personnel to help move your charge, move heavy items out of the way, or even break things to enter or exit your home. Here's how to start preparing your home.

Do a Home Walk-Through

Imagine you're an EMT or another responder walking fast, maybe even running, into your home with lots of heavy medical equipment, accompanied by a team of other responders. Ask yourself, could they find you quickly? What's in their way? What's missing? What will they need to know about?

Start your walk-through by going outside to the front of your home—in the driveway, in the parking lot, or at your building or house entrance. Bring a yardstick or measuring tape with you (you'll need it for doors and hallways). Turn around and retrace your steps inside, all the while looking at and noting everything up, down, and around you. Once inside, inspect the access ways into your home and into every room.

If you have a cell phone, or small camera, take pictures to review and make sure that pathways appear clear and safe for an emergency team to enter and get to our charge.

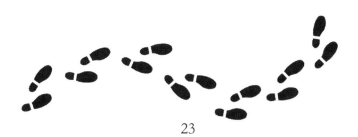

Start Outside

- ❏ Are there signs for your mailbox, street, house, building, and/or apartment, and are they well-lit with **numbers and letters clearly visible from a distance**?

- ❏ Are the numbers and letters light reflective or in a color that **contrasts from the background** they are on?

- ❏ Are the numbers and **letters large enough to be seen** easily by a passing emergency vehicle?

- ❏ Is anything **blocking the numbers and letters** from view, such as trees, bushes, other signs, construction materials, and so forth?

If your house number is missing, put up (or have someone put up) a number that's large enough, and contrasts enough, to be easily seen from the street. Many towns and jurisdictions regulate the size of house and building numbers. The size of residential home numbers usually range from three to six inches tall.

If you live in an apartment or rented home and the building numbers are missing, contact the building owners or management in writing. If street signs are missing, write to the village, town, or city. Be polite, but insistent, about safety implications. Keep dated copies of your correspondence for follow up, if needed.

Between the street/driveway and first door inside, look for anything in the way, such as lawn chairs, benches, trash cans, and other things left out that could block a stretcher or large medical equipment. This goes for building hallways to your door, too.

Move things enough so that responders can easily gain access to your home, without causing themselves injury, while still allowing you to enjoy your home.

If other people's property is in the way, politely let them know about the situation and potential risks. Most will cooperate. Those who won't cooperate should be contacted and notified of conditions in writing. Don't argue, but try to convince those who can get things fixed that safety is more important than convenience.

Moving to Your Doorway

- ❑ Is your entry door partially blocked or cluttered with boxes, kids' stuff, furniture, plants, seasonal ornaments, or other entry way hazards? ❑ Is your entry door wide enough? **Measure it**. A standard stretcher is 24 inches wide and seven feet long. Doors and hallways need to have room to swing a stretcher through. Otherwise, responders may have to use alternate equipment, which may slow them down.

    Note: *If entryways are too narrow and can't be changed, it's important to let the 911 dispatcher and responders know that, either before or as soon as they arrive.*

- ❑ Are doors set up to remain unlocked after opening? EMTs are usually not authorized to break into your home. Fire departments are equipped to enter your home, but if they need to be called in to break a door open, critical medical help could be significantly delayed.

- ❑ Are people **available to unlock doors,** including apartment buzzer systems, in an emergency?

Consider installing a **First Responder Safe Box** on the front door if someone is not always there to let responders in. This is a small combination lock box attached to the front door, holding a key or combination to your home lock. Give your local responders the combination so that they can gain access without damaging your door (or windows). Check with local authorities for how to sign up for this program, if available. Otherwise, tell the 911 dispatcher if you have one, and ask them to relay the combination to responders who need to enter your home.

As an alternative, if affordable, you can install a remote-capable electronic lock on the door. Most come with phone apps and door cameras. You should identify someone you trust to whom you can give backup access when you're not available.

Inside your home

Consider whether a stretcher can easily get up stairways, down halls, and into rooms without someone tripping or falling over cords, area rugs, or other items.

Do a visual check (with a measure), and identify and move furniture, items, and tripping hazards so that there's a clear, wide enough path (ideally, more than two feet wide with room to swing a seven-foot stretcher) for responders to easily get to your charge with their equipment.

Move or fasten down everything. Rug grip tape can be placed under the edges of area rugs to prevent them from curling up or sliding on a bare floor. Reroute extension cords out of the way. Gaffer or duct tape can be laid over exposed cords. Bright colored tape should be visibly placed to warn about steps or uneven flooring.

Is each room clearly and brightly lit? Check lights to make sure they work and are not too dim. Make sure you always have **more lights in every room than you think are necessary**. You can always turn them down or off.

Can phone(s) be reached quickly? In your charge's home, identify a location where you can always put your cell phone and will know where it is in an emergency. Keep an extra charger nearby so your phone can always stay charged and be ready to use. Know where all landlines and extensions are in the home. Landline phones should be kept in a highly visible location at all times.

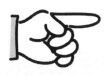
Prepare Your Home Summary

➤ Make sure responders can **easily find** and **identify your street home address** and other identifying numbers from the road, quickly. All responders have told us that this is critically important!

➤ Make sure that responders can get to the person in need **without tripping over things, having to move furniture or or even breaking doors or windows**.

➤ Now is the time to **organize, remove excess furniture and items**, and clear your home of items that have little to no personal meaning or value. Aim to create fast emergency entry and exit paths.

➤ **Note**: If some doors, stairways, and halls are not wide enough to get stretchers and equipment through quickly, **notify responders of such situations that you can't fix, either before or when they first arrive**.

➤ **Clutter tends to build up slowly.** Do a walkthrough at least every six months so you know that responders can still easily, reach, get into, and get out of your home.

Prepare Your Environment

You should gain an understanding of where all potential responders are based, what you can expect of them, and who else can help in a pinch. It's also a good idea to try to get all those who may wind up helping you to understand your specific needs and situations.

Know Your Community

Getting to know your community takes a lot more than just knowing your neighbors. Take time to locate your local police department, fire department, emergency medical responders, hospitals, emergency clinics, doctors, and other care providers and determine their accessibility in relation to your home and work. It is important to understand how long it can take for any of them to get to you and your charge in an emergency.

Identify and note where your community emergency teams are located, including:

Police Department

- ❑ Post the **local phone numbers** for the police next to or with your **File of Life** and in your cell phone contacts. This is important in case, for some reason, you can't get through to a 911 dispatcher and need immediate assistance.

- ❑ Note how far they are located from home — distance in miles and minutes at an average driving speed. This will help you estimate how quickly responders can get to you, which in turn may give you an idea of how long you will need to provide critical care before responders arrive.

- ❑ Learn what additional services are available through, or associated with, your police department. Some towns have an elderly "check-in" service where someone calls and checks on your charge daily to make sure they're safe and well. Find out if this service is available near you and how to sign up for it.

Fire Department/EMT

❑ As with the police, post the local fire department and EMT numbers next to your File of Life, in your cell phone contacts, and if you have one, near your landline phone.

Get Out and About

Visit and introduce yourself to your local emergency responders: police, fire, EMTs/paramedics. Find out who, specifically, in those departments you can meet with (and when) to discuss your homecare situations. It's best to make an appointment to speak with such personnel, especially at very busy stations.

❑ Explain who you are and tell them about your home, eldercare, or special needs situations.

❑ If available, register your charge as a person in the community who may need help being evacuated (and why) in an emergency.

❑ If you need access to an emergency power supply for life support, ask if they have a way to help you or can give advice on what to do should the power go out in your home for an extended period of time.

❑ Learn where emergency shelters are located, what is provided there, and how and when they are made available.

❑ Find out about visiting nurse and home health care type agencies that operate in your area. Learn what services they offer, and what affiliations they have with medical care facilities.

Neighbors, Friends, Family: Don't Be Shy!

For additional support, introduce yourself, ask around, and determine which of your **neighbors** would be **willing to help** you if there's an emergency. Add their phone numbers and emails to your emergency contact list. Offering to do the same for them, if you can, may make it easier.

If you have friends or family close by, start up, form, or join an informal mutual aid group. For those willing and capable of doing so, get a solid understanding of each other's family caregiving needs and who can do what in the event of an emergency. Once established and agreed upon, exchange contact information. Everyone involved should be aware of the seriousness of promising to pitch in when asked and understand how much others will rely on one another. Impress on everyone that, if there's a likelihood that **they can't help when called upon, don't volunteer.**

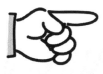# Prepare Your Environment Summary

- Know where your local **police department, fire department, emergency medical responders, and hospitals** are all located.

- Post the **local police, fire, and EMT phone numbers** next to your File of Life (in case 911 goes out).

- Visit and **introduce yourself** to your local emergency responders: police, fire, EMTs, and paramedics. Learn what additional services are available. Explain your home, elder care, or special needs situations.

- **Learn where emergency shelters and local senior centers are located**, and what they offer.

- Determine **which of your neighbors would be willing to help** you if there's an emergency.

- Start up or join an **informal mutual aid group** of willing and capable caregivers.

2

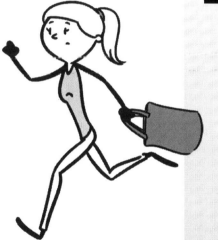

Prepare To Give Help

Prepare Everyone!

In this process, preparing to give help involves more than just having helpful things handy when needed. Once you realize that something bad has happened, it's up to you, the family caregiver, to give or get help for them.

That help may simply involve giving basic first aid: applying antibiotic and a Band-Aid, putting some cold on a bump or bruise, pulling a splinter, or wrapping a torn fingernail or toenail. Knowing how to apply first aid in emergency situations will enable you to better identify when help that is needed is beyond your ability.

In addition, once you've made that 911 call, providing needed care yourself, until responders arrive, may mean life or death to someone in desperate need. You may have to keep their heart going, keep their airway open, breathe for them, stop or slow bleeding, or get them further out of harm's way. That's when having first aid training, knowing cardiopulmonary resuscitation (CPR), knowing how to use an automated external defibrillator (AED), and having related equipment on hand become critical.

In order give help promptly until others arrive, you need to gain a pretty good understanding of what to do. That involves building up and keeping up your potentially life-saving skills. It will take commitment on your part and an investment in time, energy, and, perhaps, some funds.

The return on that investment, however, may be priceless. It all depends on what value you place on yourself and on those for whom you care.

Learn Basic First Aid

Let's repeat: *learn basic first aid.* **You can't be a good caregiver without knowing this.** Knowing first aid will come in handy even with non-emergency care for yourself and others. Knowing what to do for major health issues will help you to better cope when they occur. You'll also better understand an emergency dispatcher's instructions during a 911 call and stay focused on what you need to do, right then and there.

Learn and practice how to apply first aid in different emergency situations, such as excessive bleeding, strokes, heart attacks, falls, burns, or shock. Especially learn how to treat elderly, frail, infirm, or special needs individuals. There are three ways to get the basic first aid knowledge you need:

- ❏ In-person courses
- ❏ Online courses and videos
- ❏ Books

The *American Red Cross* and the *American Heart Association* have long, successful histories of training non-medical professionals in the basics of emergency first aid. In addition, you can often find first aid courses near you that are sponsored by a local community or government agencies, including volunteer responder groups. Fire departments, paramedics, and EMTs can also tell you where to get first aid training. These courses can typically take a few hours to a few days to complete and often include take-home instruction manuals and tip sheets for reference and to share with others.

Many first aid education courses are also available online. Some focus on the specific needs of children, adults, or the elderly. When considering any online health education, remember that classroom and one-on-one training can give you a more realistic way of seeing and experiencing what to expect in an emergency. However, online training is definitely far better than no training at all.

If you want to learn more through self-guided training, there are hundreds of first aid books and free or low-cost first aid information online. When choosing, consider books or courses that may seem to be the easiest for you to understand, such as those using non-medical language and having lots of illustrations.

Self-education can be effective, provided you stay up with new practices and applications and seek additional advice from trained medical professionals whenever possible. It's important to stay current with all information as practices, such as CPR, stroke response, and bleeding control, have been updated in recent years. The more you learn, the more likely you and yours will have positive outcomes in emergency situations.

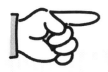
Basic First Aid Summary

- Don't wait: **take a course on basic first aid NOW**. Doing so could save your life or the life of someone who desperately needs it.

- The American Heart Association, American Red Cross, some local government agencies, community groups, and/or emergency responders often offer these courses. **Call your city or town hall, local fire department, or EMS and ask.**

- While classroom and one-on-one training may provide more realistic ways to understand how to respond to mishaps and emergencies, **online training** is far better than getting no training at all. If online courses are your only near-term option, consider taking easy-to-understand, self-guided, and structured courses.

- Get a **basic first aid book that looks easy to follow** and read it before you attend any course. **Get or make copies** to put into your first aid kits. This will help you become more informed and ready to ask questions of medical personnel about your own charge's situation.

Household First Aid Kits

Every household should have a First Aid Kit. Every house that has elderly, frail, or infirm individuals, or those who need specialized assistance, should consider having a more personalized First Aid Kit. Such kits serve as a handy resource for treating minor conditions, pain, and injuries from mishaps, illnesses, and household accidents. More importantly, they can be used for interim treatment for emergencies until more help arrives.

Your First Aid Kit should be organized around potential issues and for the specific needs of those in the household. Here's a way to build your own household's first aid kit, with some special considerations for the elderly and infirmed.

Start by gathering together, then laying out everything that should go into your kit. When you've collected everything, you can then decide how big a box or bag you'll need to hold everything, with room for additional items as conditions change. It should be sturdy enough to last going through again and again. It doesn't need to be fancy, but you should be able to retrieve most things inside without pulling everything out of the kit.

Clearly mark the outside front, back, and sides of your kit in large red lettering as "First Aid' or with a big red-colored cross. You should be able to quickly identify a First Aid Kit in a dark, dimly lit, or crowded closet or spot. Always store your kit where you can get to it in a few seconds. Faster responses improve the likelihood of better outcomes.

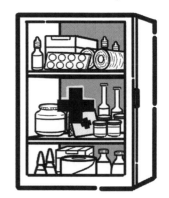

Items to consider for a household First Aid Kit include:

- One small flashlight (attached to outside of bag/box); headband/hands-free type flashlights can be more convenient
- Three permanent pen/markers.
    - Two VERY large red and black, 1/2 inch wide or more
    - One writing felt tip pen
- 25 to 50 various sized, sensitive skin adhesive bandages (small to extra-large); Nexcare brand has several sizes for delicate and fragile skin
- Ten individual Steri-strip type adhesive wound closures
- One DermaFilm type bandage or a moisture-vapor permeable dressing
- One large, resealable or tie-up plastic bag (to use for contaminated waste)
- One to two paper lunch bags (help with hyperventilation)
- One small box of paper napkins or tissues
- One small bottle of anesthetic spray
- Two small, sealed hand sanitizer bottles
- One tube hydrocortisone ointment
- One tube barrier cream
- One dental kit (for broken/lost teeth)
- One eyewash kit
- Ingrown toenail file
- Antifungal foot powder
- Epsom Salt
- One small box cotton swabs
- Two rolls of elastic bandages (Ace type, large and small)

- ☐ One small bottle of saline water
- ☐ One small jar petroleum jelly
- ☐ One magnifying glass
- ☐ Five 5 x 9 inch absorbent compress bandage dressings
- ☐ One roll of adhesive cloth tape (10 yards x one inch)
- ☐ Ten antibiotic ointment packets or one tube of triple antibiotic ointment
- ☐ 20 antiseptic wipe packages (large size)
- ☐ One foil thermal blanket (space blanket)
- ☐ One soft, thin roll-up pillow
- ☐ One CPR breathing barrier (with a one-way valve)
- ☐ One tube of Burn Jel or Water Jel type burn ointment to cool and soothe
- ☐ One pair of blunt nose, right angle scissors
- ☐ Two gauze bandage rolls, three inches wide
- ☐ Two gauze bandage rolls, four inches wide
- ☐ 10 sterile gauze pads (four x four inches square)
- ☐ Two packs of sterile cotton lint-free pads for wound care
- ☐ Three to five instant cold compresses
- ☐ Three to five instant hot compresses
- ☐ One digital thermometer, or ten thermometer strips
- ☐ Two tweezers: round nose and pointed nose
- ☐ Five-plus untreated oral foam swab sticks
- ☐ Four pairs of non-latex gloves (large)
- ☐ Four packs of aspirin and acetaminophen (or small bottles)

- ❏ Two triangular bandages
- ❏ First aid instruction book
- ❏ Ammonia inhalants

Customize the First Aid Kit by including items that could be useful for those in the household with special needs, such as:

- ❏ Celox or Wound Seal packets (quick clotting powder)
- ❏ EpiPen (with prescription) or fast release antihistamine
- ❏ Naloxone (Narcan) nasal spray (may require a prescription)
- ❏ Pulse oximeter
- ❏ Portable blood pressure cuff
- ❏ Glucose meter

Some of these may require prescriptions and will need periodic updates and maintenance.

It may not be practical to store some often-used items in the First Aid kit. Example, the blood pressure cuff and the pulse oximeter.

Check your First Aid Kit contents at least once every three months to make sure that no item has gone bad or passed its expiration date. Write your last inspection date on a card and place in the kit.

After each use, do an inventory and refresh, refill, replace, or add new useful items so the kit is ready and fully stocked for the next use or emergency. Add items that could have been useful if you had them during the last emergency.

The above checklist is only basic. Each household needs to consider what special-needs items to add and keep in their First Aid Kit.

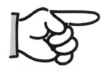

First Aid Kit Summary

- ➢ Keep a small, powerful **flashlight** attached to the side, or just inside, your First Aid Kit.

- ➢ Keep the First Aid Kit stored where you can **easily get to** it in an emergency, even in the dark.

- ➢ Take an **inventory** of its contents at least every three months and **restock**, **update**, and **replace** items used.

- ➢ **Add specific items** beyond the basics that may be beneficial to your charge's **specific needs**. For example: EpiPens, catheters, compression socks, glucose, oxygen, or pulse meters, etc. Naloxone (Narcan) should be considered for inclusion in the kit when anyone in the household is taking opioids.

- ➢ Place a note near or inside your File of Life, **reminding everyone in your home where the household First Aid Kit is located**, and when it was last inventoried.

Learn How to do CPR and Use an AED

Knowing how to give CPR could mean the difference between life and death for someone who may need it. Knowing how to conduct CPR on all body types can raise a caregiver's confidence in managing heart-related emergency calls almost anywhere they may happen.

Knowing how and when to properly conduct CPR on frail or elderly persons is even more important, since their bodies can be easily damaged. CPR, done properly, requires continued deep chest compressions. When conducting CPR on someone whose bones may be brittle, one can crack ribs, cause internal bleeding, or create other life-threatening injuries.

CPR training is often paired with AED training. An AED is used to help those in cardiac arrest. It is an easy-to-use, yet advanced medical device that can analyze the heart's rhythm and deliver, if needed, an electrical shock (defibrillation) to help re-establish an effective heart rhythm. It's important to know how and when to use both CPR and an AED.

CPR/AED skills, besides being critically useful, can help you remain calm and in control during frightening and chaotic events. These potentially life-saving skills, which can be learned from a variety of sources, are what all good caregivers should master and maintain through regular practice.

AEDs are becoming quite commonplace. While there is no federal requirement for placement in buildings, most states have requirements for having AEDs in places of public accommodation (malls, gyms, churches, offices, etc.).

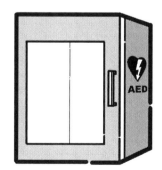

In addition, virtually all ambulances and many first responder vehicles will have these devices on board. Being able to safely use an AED can prove invaluable in administering timely, life-saving aid to a heart attack victim, whether for your charge, a family member, or even a stranger in desperate need.

Register for and attend a local CPR/AED course. Such courses may be available through:

- ❑ The **American Heart Association**
- ❑ The **American Red Cross**
- ❑ The **American CPR Care Association**
- ❑ Your local EMS, fire department, senior center, and adult education and community groups
- ❑ Online (if nothing else is available or affordable)

AEDs for the Home

Almost everyone is at risk for a sudden cardiac arrest, even healthy persons with no history of heart issues. Having an AED, especially for those with heart issues or for those who live in remote locations, would ideally make sense. However, some serious considerations must be weighed in making such a decision. First, there is a vast array of such devices to choose from, although most work pretty much the same way. Second, the cost, at an average of $1,200 or more, may be well beyond the reach of many households, especially since many insurance plans won't cover them. Third, is the need to keep them safe from environmental extremes, ready to use, and easy to find. Fourth, each member of the household should be trained in how and when to use the device.

These factors can make the decision for having a home or personal AED for those at lower risk a complicated one.

CPR Boards

In homes that are mostly carpeted, or have heavy rugs, or where a person can't be removed safely from a bed, it may be a good idea to get a CPR Board and learn how to use it. Such devices can provide a firm surface on which to conduct CPR. If needed, you can purchase a professional grade CPR Board, improvise, or make one yourself.

- ❏ You can **buy** CPR Boards online or at medical supply stores and some pharmacies.

- ❏ You can **improvise** by using a very large, 1/2-inch thick plastic kitchen cutting board to provide support.

- ❏ You can **make a CPR Board** out of standard 1/2-inch plywood. Ask your local hardware store to cut a 1/2-inch plywood or hardwood board to a dimension of 18 x 24 inches. Sand all edges so they are smooth, splinter-free, and won't cause harm when slid under someone before applying CPR. Paint or spray paint the board in a gloss finish if you can. Wax and polish are also good ideas. A smooth surface makes it easier to slide under someone when needed.

No matter how you get it, print large letters in marker or paint, on both sides of the board, "CPR." Store in a location where your charge spends most of their time (e.g., under a bed, chair, sofa, etc.).

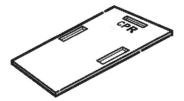

CPR training dolls can help you practice, with or without partners. CPR training equipment can be purchased, sometimes inexpensively, from a number of sources (medical supply stores, eBay, and other online marketplaces). Don't overlook "used and serviceable" for brand new equipment if it will work just as well.

Regularly, but carefully, review and practice your CPR procedures with others who've been trained so that your skills become your natural way to respond in an emergency.

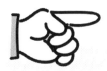

CPR and AED Summary

- ➤ Enroll in and **take a certified CPR/AED** course. Repeat as recommended, typically every two to three years.

- ➤ **Learn how to use an AED**. AEDs are becoming more and more common in public accommodating buildings.

- ➤ **If you look like you know what you're doing**, others will more likely offer to help and follow your directions.

- ➤ Mark on your calendar dates and times you will practice your CPR skills. **Practice at least four times a year** so that your skills become automatic in an emergency.

- ➤ **Keep a CPR Board** where your charge sleeps or where it can be quickly reached.

3

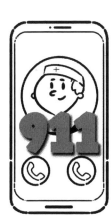

Getting Help

Getting Help From 911

In an Emergency, Dial 911 or Your Local Emergency Number Immediately!

An emergency is any situation that requires immediate assistance from the police, fire department, or medical responders. Examples include: fires; crimes, especially those in progress; car crashes, particularly if someone may be injured; and medical emergencies, especially for those needing immediate medical attention.

If you're not sure whether the situation is a true emergency, officials recommend calling 911 and letting the dispatcher determine whether you need emergency help.

A call to 911 is *not* for someone in need of companionship, non-urgent advice, referral to other services (water leaks, dead car batteries, dogs barking, noisy neighbors, etc.), or things that can be easily treated at home, in a doctor's office, or left to heal on their own. Using the 911 system to make non-urgent calls may prevent responders from caring for those in real life-threatening situations. Also, it is illegal in most places.

First Thing to Do

Keep your head! Even if your heart is racing, it's important to stop, take a deep breath, get yourself together, and carry on. This is among the most important things you can do as a caregiver.

Keep your patience as a lot of activity will occur around you. A lot will likely happen: many people may arrive (EMT, police, and maybe even firefighters), each will ask many questions, and a number of those questions will be asked repeatedly. Focus on your charge and what's happening or just happened and move forward to do what you need to do next.

Just Before Calling 911

Quickly assess the situation. Is it a **medical, fire, police-related**, or other type of emergency? Jot things down quickly, if you can, so that you don't forget, in a panic, what happened. **Have all the right information ready**. Seconds matter once the call is made.

Calling 911

If your call is not picked up immediately, do NOT hang up and try again! Stay on the line. Retrying will delay your ability to reach an emergency dispatcher. If the 911 system is busy, your call will be automatically routed to the nearest dispatcher available to help you with your emergency.

If you are put on hold: DO NOT HANG UP! Stay as patient as possible. Hanging up will put you at the back end of the phone queue and delay getting help.

Speaking with the Dispatcher (Land Line)

Dial 911. Speak slowly, clearly, and directly into your phone.

- ❑ **First tell the emergency dispatcher which type of emergency you think you have: medical, fire, police**. Example: "I have someone here who's passed out, won't wake up, and needs medical help."

- ❑ **Tell them your location**: use the exact address — street, number, apartment, etc. If you don't know, give landmarks and estimated distances from places nearby. If you're not sure, and someone, other than the person in distress, is with you, have them check the street number, street name, or other landmarks for you.

- ☐ **Tell them who you are and who needs assistance**. Describe the person's condition and age. Describe what you've done so far to help.

- [ ] Let the dispatcher guide the conversation forward from that point on. The emergency 911 dispatcher is trained to help you deal with the situation until help arrives.

- [ ] If you are physically able, after dialing 911, **put your phone in speaker mode so your hands are free** to continue any necessary care. If you are with others while providing needed care, ask them to dial for you, but ask to speak to the dispatcher directly yourself. Try not to relay information through others.

- [ ] Ask for an approximate arrival time for responders.

- [ ] If instructed by the dispatcher, and you haven't already done so, start providing CPR or first aid.

Never hang up until told to do so by responders!

Calling 911 on a Cell Phone

Dialing 911 from a cell/mobile phone adds work for an emergency dispatcher and can cause delays in getting responders to your location. Landline numbers are identified by specific location (state, city/town, and address). Your cell phone travels with you. As such, your location will change based on where your phone is at any given time. Dispatchers can only identify your location in relation to the nearest cell phone tower to you. With this in mind, how you make a 911 call on your cell phone is slightly different from using a landline.

Speaking with the Dispatcher

Dial 911. Speak slowly, clearly, and directly into your phone receiver.

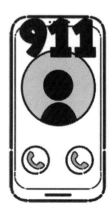

- [ ] **First tell the 911 dispatcher you're calling from a cell phone.**

- ❏ **Then tell them your location**: the exact address, street, number, apartment, etc. If you don't know, give landmarks and estimated distances from places nearby. If someone, other than the person in distress, is with you, have them check the street number, street name, or other landmarks for you.

- ❏ **Next, tell the emergency dispatcher which type of emergency you think you have: medical, fire, police.** Example: "I have someone here who has passed out, won't wake up, and needs medical help."

- ❏ **Tell them who you are and who needs assistance.** Describe the person's condition and age. Describe what you've done so far to help.

- ❏ Let the dispatcher guide the conversation forward from that point on. The emergency 911 dispatcher is trained to help you deal with the situation until help arrives.

- ❏ If you are physically able, after dialing 911, **put your phone in speaker mode** so your hands are free to continue giving necessary care. If with others, while you are providing needed care, ask them to dial for you, but ask to speak to the dispatcher yourself. Try not to relay information through another person.

- ❏ Ask for an approximate arrival time for responders.

- ❏ If instructed by the dispatcher, and you haven't already done so, start providing whatever care you know, such as CPR or first aid.

For those who care for the elderly or sensitive: you can ask the dispatcher to ask responders **not to have lights and sirens going when they arrive**. If your charge is **not in immediate danger**, you can also ask the responders to keep lights and sirens off on the way to the hospital. They will, however, turn them on if necessary when leaving your home or while in transit. Try not to get upset if this happens. Responders want to get your charge to the emergency department as soon as possible in critical emergency situations.

Never hang up until told to do so by responders!

Additional 911 Notes

If you are alone and need help, **never be afraid to call 911 for your own emergency**. Responders will work to keep you calm and get needed medical help to you as quick as they can.

The *In Case of Emergency* entry on your cell phone should **always be kept current**. Many phones have an emergency call section that responders can access without needing your password. If need be, they should be able to easily identify who you wish to have called in an emergency, if you're not capable of calling on your own. If you do not have a cell/mobile phone with this feature, tape or place your emergency contacts on a slip of paper on the back of your phone or keep it between the case and your phone.

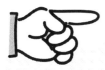

Calling 911 Summary

- When calling 911, know what to do differently when using a cell phone versus a landline.

- Always tell the dispatcher what type of emergency you think you have.

- State who needs help, who you are, what's happened, and what's been done so far.

- Give your location with as many details as possible.

- Never hang up if placed on hold.

- Follow all the dispatcher's instructions. Don't hang up until responders arrive or you are told to do so.

- If you're not getting through to the 911 dispatcher, use another phone, or get someone else to try a non-emergency contact number for fire/police/EMT.

- Whenever you can, use your speaker phone mode to free up your hands for other tasks.

Helping Out

Before Help Arrives

Make sure your **entry door is unlocked**, and stays unlocked, so that responders can quickly and easily gain entry to help you and yours. If possible, leave the door open or ajar.

- ❑ Make sure there is a **clear**, **wide**, and **easy path** for them to get to the person who needs their help. If the entry or path to your charge is cluttered, get someone to move toys, furniture, or whatever items are blocking the way.

- ❑ If you are with others, ask them to do this while you focus on the needs of your charge.

When Help Arrives

When the emergency response team arrives at your door, and you can't go to meet them personally, **yell loud and clearly**, "Come in. We're over here in the _____ room to your right (or left)." Be as specific as possible. Keep talking until they find you.

When They Reach Your Charge

- ❑ **Quickly tell the responders what's happened**, in detail. They may ask you for more information about the person in need. Remain calm and answer their questions, in the order they ask. Responders have developed procedures in how they do their work. Their job is to help your charge and you.

- ❑ **Give a copy of the injured person's File of Life to the responders.** They will later give this information to the doctors once they arrive at the hospital. This information will save time and allow them and hospital staff to more quickly assess your charge's situation and the type of care they will need.

- ❑ **Be patient**: you may be asked the same questions repeatedly and by different responders.

- ❑ **Step away and let the responders take over**: let them to do their job!

- ❑ **Retrieve, and keep near you, your charge's Go Bag** that contains all the necessary medical, legal, and personal information for your charge.

- ❑ **Call those who need to know (family, neighbors, etc.) that your charge is going to the hospital.** If you plan to go and you need help at home, or at the hospital, now is the time to ask.

- ❑ **Place your purse, wallet, phone, keys, and Go Bag in one location** so that you can quickly grab and take them with you to the hospital.

Notes for Parents and Pet Owners

Children can be easily disturbed by emergency events and can **seriously hamper** responders' abilities to provide aid. Make sure that you or someone (other than the responders) can keep children safely out of the way. It also helps to have adults keep them company to reduce their fears.

Pets can get upset too. They can easily distract, interfere with, or injure you, responders, or others — or be injured themselves during an emergency. Place pets where they can be safely kept out of the way of responders.

You should always have a plan in place and people available to take care of children and household pets during the course of an emergency.

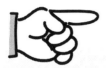

Helping Out Summary

> ➤ Once they arrive, give responders a calm, quick assessment of the situation. **Give them your charge's File of Life** as soon as you can.

> ➤ **Be patient** if the same questions are asked repeatedly. Responders follow their training and specific routines for a reason.

> ➤ Then, **step out of their way**. Trust them, and allow them to them to take control of the situation.

> ➤ **Stay nearby** by so you can answer any of the responder's questions that might help them better assess and assist your charge.

> ➤ **Keep children and pets safely away** from responders.

> ➤ Get your Go Bag, and anything else that you need, to be ready to take with you to the hospital.

> ➤ **Make arrangements for securing the household** and caring for any other occupants (other charges, children, pets, etc.) if you intend to leave.

What to do Before the Ambulance Leaves

Make sure you have everything you need ready to take with you to help those at the hospital who will be caring for your charge. Do you have the:

❑ Address and directions to the hospital?

❑ Go Bag?

❑ File of Life copies in the bag?

❑ Keys, wallet, purse, cell phone, and charger?

❑ Go Bag comfort items (if helpful to your charge)?

❑ Notebook/journal and pen?

❑ All the contact numbers that you'll need?

When the Responders Are Ready, and Before They Leave for the Hospital

If you are going with them in the ambulance:*

❑ Ask responders which hospital they will be going to. If your charge has a specific hospital by choice or necessity, be sure to let the ambulance crew know. (Note: You can ask, but they may not give you a choice.)

❑ Make sure the home will be secure and those left behind will remain safe.

❑ Contact those who need to know what's happened, and tell them where you are going.

❑ Call on your support group to help out while you're gone with your charge.

- ❑ Take all the things you've put out (purse/wallet, keys, phone, and Go Bag).

- ❑ Stay out of the way. Follow all instructions you are given by the responders once your charge is in the ambulance.

- ❑ Ask about how to make arrangements to get yourself and your charge back home from the hospital. The ambulance may not be able to return you home when you want.

- * *Many ambulance crews won't allow you to ride with them to the hospital unless you are a parent or special needs caregiver.*

If you plan to follow the ambulance to the hospital:

- ❑ Ask responders **which hospital or facility they will be going to**. Get the address of the hospital before they leave with your charge. Enter the address in your phone GPS or get directions.

- ❑ Make sure the home and those left behind will remain safe.

- ❑ Drive to the hospital emergency department calmly and safely. Don't block any entrances or take up any official or assigned spaces when parking.

If you cannot go to the hospital with your charge because you have another person or child to care for at home:

- ❑ Call a friend, co-worker, or family member and ask if they can come to your home to mind other occupants while you go to the hospital. If no one is available, take the others with you to the hospital, if feasible.

- ❑ Otherwise, you may have to wait near your phone, while you send someone you trust to go in your place, along with your charge's Go Bag, after giving them instructions on what's in there and how to use it.

When you arrive at the hospital:

❑ Go immediately to the hospital's emergency department.

❑ Tell the front or admissions desk that your charge has arrived at the hospital via ambulance.

❑ Tell them that you have all medical records and other important files with you, in case they require them.

❑ If your charge is not in an immediate life-threatening situation, ask to be escorted to see your charge. If you explain that you have important information for their use, this may happen more quickly.

Note: If you are male, and your charge (or spouse) is female, you may be separated from her by hospital staff for some time while they assess her health and well-being. This is typically done because they may want to determine if physical or spousal abuse caused the medical emergency. Understand that this is a very real issue. Try to avoid feeling insulted or getting more upset. With abuse cases increasing in the United States, this type of questioning process has become part of many hospital emergency departments' protocols. It should not be thought of as a bad thing for them to do.

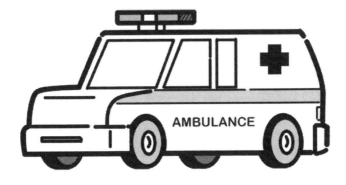

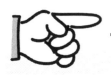

What to Do When The Ambulance Leaves Summary

- If your charge is unconscious, or not able to make their own decisions, responders will make their own decision as to whether to take them to the hospital.

- Ambulance transport may have costs. While often covered by insurance, ambulance transport or medical airlifting can be very costly.

- **You can refuse to have your charge transported by ambulance** if you are authorized to make informed decisions for your charge and have other means to get your charge to a hospital. You are then **taking all the risks** in getting your charge there safely. However, you need to understand that **ambulance arrivals get top priority at any hospital**.

- Get the name and address of the hospital where your charge will be taken. Write down and enter the address or put in your cell phone for your GPS.

- Call those who can help you care for those who can't be left at home alone.

- Notify those who need to know about the situation and how to reach you.

- Make sure your house, other occupants, pets, and so forth will remain safe and secure if you leave.

- When you arrive at the hospital, bring all relevant medical information to the emergency department, admittance, or front desk personnel.

At the Hospital Emergency Department

Those who arrive at the hospital by ambulance or emergency vehicle almost always get a faster response from medical staff. Ambulance arrivals are presumed by the hospital to need immediate medical care.

If you walk into a hospital emergency department on your own with an urgent issue, **you may not get attention right away**, even if you say you're having a heart attack.

First, you need to understand some **Basic Trigger Words** that may get you more attention right at the admissions desk. If you walk in and are in bad shape, you should loudly state (and if necessary, yell out) to the admitting staff what the specific problem is that needs immediate help: "I (CAN'T BREATHE or AM ABOUT TO PASS OUT or HE'S HAVING REALLY BAD CHEST PAINS or HE CAN'T STOP BLEEDING or SHE CAN'T SEE or I CAN'T FEEL MY FACE/ARMS/LEGS or I HAVE THE WORST HEAD PAIN OF MY LIFE, etc.) and NEED HELP NOW!" Don't be shy! This may get you faster attention.

- ❑ Give the admitting personnel a copy of your charge's File of Life. This improves the likelihood of your charge receiving faster attention than those who don't arrive with detailed medical information.

- ❑ Tell the admitting nurse or doctor of any other medical conditions about your charge that may not be covered in the File of Life.

- ❑ Relate the details of what happened, why you called 911, and why you are at the emergency department. For example:

    - Explain charge's symptoms

- When those symptoms started
- How long the symptoms have persisted
- Any changes in the symptoms since they started, and
- What might have caused the symptoms, if you know (don't guess).

❑ What you did to help your charge before you called 911, and have done before responders arrived.

❑ If requested, now is the time to give them what they ask for from the Go Bag. Once your charge is in the medical team's care, you may be asked for:

- Insurance cards/information
- Other legal and medical information and copies of medical directives/DNR, POLSTs, living wills, guardianship, etc.
- The POA for the person if they are unable to make their own decisions.

Note: *Once a child is of legal age (18 in most states), parents will not be able to gain access to their medical records legally unless they are their legal guardians, have a POA, or have children who are not mentally or physically capable of making decisions themselves. You will not be able to get access to medical updates unless you have a POA or are a designated guardian or spouse and have adequate proof.*

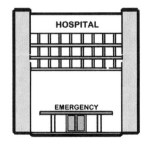

Once in the Emergency Department

Once your charge is in the emergency department, your objective is to try to get them evaluated and treated as soon as possible. In a notebook, write down the time that you and your charge entered the emergency department.

In a busy emergency department, your charge can easily be overlooked or mistakenly forgotten. Make sure your charge has an identifier on them at all times (bracelet, sticky note, anything will do at first) with their name and date of birth noted, at minimum. This could be on a hospital supplied band. You can also safety pin the information on their clothing somewhere. Or, in a pinch, write their name and date of birth right on their (good) lower arm or leg with a felt tip marker.

Once Treatment Is Underway

Always know where your charge is in the emergency department and where they will be taken to for evaluation, tests, or emergency treatment. Bad things can happen when a patient is left outside a testing location without a family member, someone familiar, or medical personnel at their side.

Don't be shy! Find out, as soon as possible, and write down the name of the doctor in charge of the emergency department shift. Next, get and write down the name of the attending doctor for your charge. Then learn the name of the nurses/technicians handling your charge's care. Write all of their names down, too. Make note of every person who comes in to speak with or attend to your charge.

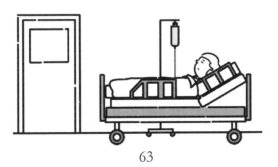

Speak directly to those assigned to your charge's care when they are freed up and appear available to speak with you. Ask about:

- ❑ Your charge's state of condition
- ❑ Tests being or planning to be performed and results from any that were done
- ❑ Decisions on what they will do next and what may need to be decided by you, and/or the medical team, about your charge's care/treatment
- ❑ The expected length of time in the emergency department
- ❑ Plans to admit your charge and specific hospital admission procedures.

Note: *If your charge is to be admitted under observation, get a full understanding of how or whether your insurance will cover it.*

Patients who are admitted under observation can experience major financial implications. **Many insurance plans do not cover the cost of admission under observation. On the reverse side, under certain plans, being admitted under observation can be less costly than full admission.**

Have the hospital recheck with your charge's insurance provider details regarding which admission procedures are (or are not) covered. If your charge's insurance does not cover one or the other, insist that your charge be admitted with full consideration for your charge's best insurance coverage and financial situation.

Note: *If you don't get answers, be polite (emergency department medical personnel can often get overwhelmed), but be persistent. You came to the emergency department for a reason and deserve answers — even if not right away. Getting to know who is who and who is in charge can go a long way to getting you what you need to know.*

Special Considerations for Elderly Patients

Hospital emergency departments have their ebb and flow and may seem chaotic to outsiders. Emergency departments have specific procedures for how to respond to various emergency situations. They often deal with multiple, concurrent stressful emergency situations and may not give you or your charge the time or attention you think you need or deserve. The attention of emergency department doctors, nurses, and other medical staff are fully focused on saving the lives of those who come before them.

When your charge is stabilized, some medical staff who come to their side may not realize your charge has a hearing, sight, or memory-loss condition. They may start asking questions or providing diagnoses or medical opinions quickly and bluntly. Being there at the side of your charge will help ease some confusion or distress if the medical team inadvertently causes it.

Special considerations to note include:

❑ If your charge is hard of hearing, make sure the doctor speaks slowly, clearly, and directly to them.

- Repeat the questions for your charge or answer any questions for them that they can't hear or answer directly.

- If necessary, tactfully remind staff to treat your charge with the same respect given to anyone with full physical and mental capacities.

❑ If you believe that the medical staff thinks your charge has dementia, Alzheimer's, or a mental impairment **and you know that they do not have such a condition or affliction**:

- Tactfully tell them that your charge has full cognitive capabilities, but they may simply be hard of hearing, temporarily disoriented, or unable to fully comprehend the language or accent spoken, etc.

- If your charge does have dementia, Alzheimer's, or a mental impairment, make sure that medical staff don't talk over or about your charge as if they were not in the room. Ask the medical staff to include them in the conversation with you. Doing so will help them understand what's happening, and let them feel that they are in good care.

☐ Do not leave your charge's side, unless they are being taken to another area of the hospital for tests.

- Ask if it is possible for you to follow and, if needed, hold their hand or stay close while they're being wheeled to a different room for tests.

- Be attentive or keep your charge calm and comfortable during any test or, at least, wait just outside the testing room door. Explain that this will give your charge some comfort in being with someone familiar, and in knowing they are not alone.

☐ Make sure that your charge's possessions are safely stored where they will not be lost or stolen.

☐ Items get lost in hospitals. Some hospitals now have security personnel in the emergency department to document and, if necessary, safely secure all personal items. This includes cell phones, laptops and tablets, purses and wallets, glasses, clothing, keys, accessories, jewelry, watches, or other items that your charge has with them when they arrive at the emergency department.

- If your charge is wearing jewelry or has any other valuable possessions—financial or sentimental—ask if you can help them remove the items so that you can keep them safe.

☐ Keep a notebook or journal, and pen with you at all times.

- Take notes on conversations with the medical staff and document their answers to your questions. This includes questions or conversations that you may not completely understand or comprehend. Include notes on what the doctors and staff say about potential side effects or medical outcomes of procedures and tests.

- Restate your understanding after situations and expected outcomes are shared with you. Confirm with medical staff whether your understanding is correct or not. Ask them to review your notes and correct any misunderstandings.

This information will be helpful later if or when you relay your charge's condition, treatment, and prognoses to others.

A Note About Hospital-Induced Delirium

Delirium is a condition that shows up as sudden changes in a patient's mental state. This can include symptoms such as confusion, agitation, hallucinations, withdrawal, anger and aggression (verbal and physical), and lack of inhibition. Some refer to it as Sundowner's Syndrome (as it often happens near sundown or in the evening hours). On the flip side, it can evolve with such symptoms as withdrawal, disinterest, and even unresponsiveness.

Hospital-induced delirium is not a rare occurrence, yet it is often missed by hospital staff. The condition can progress and result in serious consequences. It's more common in the elderly, those with some mental impairment, and the terminally ill, **but anyone hospitalized (and at any age) can be at risk**.

There can be a number of triggers, some made in combination, that prompt this condition while being treated. These may include unfamiliar surroundings and faces, the routines of hospital staff, the time of day, and the reason the patient came in (overdose, failure to take medications, pain, urinary tract infection, septicemia, physical trauma, fatigue, etc.).

Since delirium often mimics dementia, some hospitals will medicate those showing agitation or anxiety. Sometimes those treatments can make the condition a lot worse. What do you do if these symptoms show up in your charge?

- First, **keep your head**.
- **Be aware** of what may be going on.
- **Be vocal**: let hospital staff know the situation is not typical behavior in your charge.
- **Be an advocate**: ask for changes in some hospital routines that can cause unnecessary disturbances (too much noise, light, multiple blood pressure or blood tests at night, etc.), and question the need for sedatives and other drugs that haven't been used before.
- **Bring familiar things**: consider bringing glasses, hearing aids, and items that normally comfort a patient while at home.
- Finally, **be there** or have someone stay there to reassure them as much as possible!

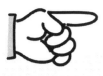
Emergency Department Summary

- If you walk into the emergency department with your own life-threatening medical emergency, loudly state, or even yell that you need help RIGHT NOW and name the type of emergency you're having. Do not worry how you sound or be embarrassed.

- If possible, **always bring your Go Bag** with an additional copy of all necessary medical and insurance information.

- Give a copy of the relevant information from your Go Bag to administrators, medical staff, and/or anyone in a position of treatment authority if they request it.

- Stay out of everyone's way whenever treatment is being applied. Let the emergency department staff know where you will be if you leave the department temporarily (restroom, cafeteria, car, lobby, etc.).

- Ask for updates on admission, condition, tests, and medical care decisions.

- Don't interfere with emergency department doctors or staff operations, **but don't be afraid to be persistent in asking** if you don't get answers to your questions.

4

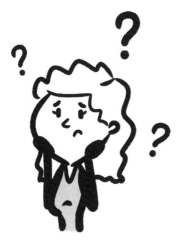

What's Next

What's Next

For Your Charge

After the emergency, there is always the question of "what's next" for your charge, and you. Everyone may need to adjust to a "new normal." However, when caring for an older, frail, or more infirm person after an emergency, daily care needs, routines, and procedures are much more likely to shift. You should always push for an honest and direct opinion on your charge's current condition and prognosis for the future from the discharge doctor.

When it's time for your charge to be discharged from the hospital, medical professionals may recommend that care be continued, either temporarily or permanently, at one of the following locations:

- ❏ **Home**, with no changes to care, or new or increased levels or types of care
- ❏ A temporary care-type facility, such as a **skilled nursing** or a **rehabilitation facility**
- ❏ A custodial-type care facility, such as a **nursing home**, **assisted living facility**, or **memory care unit or facility**
- ❏ **Hospice care** at home or in a facility for hospice care

Giving or getting care at each of these locations may differ substantially and require additional preparations, different caring skills, medical equipment, and/or new specialized medical services to treat your charge.

Getting Discharged From the Hospital

The time it takes hospital personnel to discharge someone from the hospital can take hours, involve multiple hospital departments, and be frustrating for you and your charge. Unfortunately, this is not a part of the overall emergency care process that you want to skip. Discharge doesn't mean you are at the end of the emergency. Think of it as a new starting point for you and your charge to understand why the emergency occurred and how to move on or into a new phase of care.

If you are having difficulty getting discharge papers for your charge, here are some suggestions for speeding up the process:

- ❑ Check and double check insurance information and reconfirm what was discussed during the admissions process.

- ❑ Get a clear understanding of the hospital's discharge process, paperwork, and required authorizations, as several departments may be involved.

- ❑ Ask for the name of the doctor responsible for personally signing discharge forms.

- ❑ Be prepared to run errands and pick up papers for signatures if needed, if that's what it takes to move things along.

- ❑ Frequently ask for details along the way on where things are in the process.

- ❑ Get/pickup discharge medications from the hospital pharmacy ahead of time and inform appropriate discharge personnel that you have these items in hand.

- ❑ Make a plan for getting your charge to their next location. The hospital will want to know your plans for getting your charge home or to another place for continued care. Hospitals may seriously delay discharge if they don't believe your charge will be transported safely. If you don't have these plans clearly laid out, ask for suggestions.

❏ Ask to speak with the next level of authority if you get stuck. That may be the hospital head nurse, attending physician, or hospital administration.

Discharge Documents

It is possible for you (if you have the POA for your charge) or your charge to seek a hospital discharge at any time, but it's not always the best decision, even if the long wait may make it appealing.

Each hospital has its own discharge policies. If you choose to follow them, it will mean obtaining, reading, and understanding the hospital's discharge documents (i.e., papers, summaries, etc.).

Have all documents printed out for you to read and review. If you do not agree with some of the contents, cross out, initial, and date the points that you do not agree to (this is why you get a printed copy). **Be very careful about signing anything electronically, as you may not be able to alter electronic documents**. Going through this step may delay your charge's discharge, but if you do not agree with items in those documents, you should question and/or note your disagreement to those points.

Take additional time to review all documents with the discharge person. Make sure that you fully understand all instructions, medications, side effects, complications that might arise, and what changes (if any) to look for in your charge.

Be sure to discuss any reasonable alternatives to recommendations for continued care, treatments, and rehabilitation at facilities as compared to in-home care and/or therapy. Ask for details on why they were prescribed and potential side effects or complications that you should look for. Do not worry about how much of their time you are taking during this process. It is their job to make sure you fully comprehend all aspects of the discharge documents and related recommendations.

Also, understand the legal and financial ramifications of what you're agreeing to in all signed documents. For example, if you are not personally responsible for covering your charge's finances (out of your own pocket), make sure you are not volunteering to assume responsibility for any hospital charges. Take notes, and if you do not understand, ask!

Getting to Where You're Going

No matter where your charge will be going after discharge, you will need to make sure they can get safely home or to their new or temporary facility. If you are not able to do so safely, the hospital will strongly discourage releasing them.

If you need medical transport, the hospital can help you with selecting and ordering safe transportation for your charge.

There are many more details that you'll need to consider if you have to quickly select a facility for your charge. There are more scenarios than we can cover in this book. The hospital discharge personnel, if asked, will likely be able to direct, and help you with the selection of a facility.

The following offers some information to consider when faced with certain discharge options that you might not already be familiar with.

Discharged to Home

Before you've been told officially that your charge can leave the hospital, get a full understanding of what you may need to do to make changes, if any, to make the home, safe, secure, and comfortable. This should also make caregiving easier.

Medical emergencies can be stressful to everyone involved, including both charge and caregiver. The first day or two at home will likely take some re-adjustment. You and your charge may be fatigued. Don't push things. You will both likely need to get some extra rest and sleep.

If no changes to your charge's care at home were recommended, it's still important to get an understanding as to why the emergency may have happened in the first place and what, if anything, can be done to prevent a recurrence.

If changes were recommended, such as new medical equipment, follow-up care, or permanent medical attention, make the necessary adjustments to your home and arrangements to get the required new aid or support as soon as you can. Then, when things are in order, you and your charge should work to rest and recover.

If you need an extra hand in caring for your charge, or you just need a break, call family, friends, or neighbors (maybe that mutual support network you've been working on) for a few hours of their time. If you can get a friend, companion, or a health care aide to help, a few hours off for you will be a blessing to your own health and well-being.

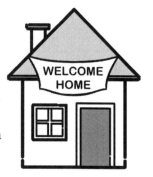

If you need to, hire a home health care aide or someone to help with household chores and companionship for your charge. Check with Medicare or your charge's insurance carrier or long-term care policy for what's covered or reimbursable.

If you need it, before discharge is complete, ask the hospital's social worker or discharge staff for recommendations on where to find private care nurses, Home Health Aides (HHA), Certified Nursing Assistants (CNA), other type of home health care specialists, housekeeping support, an agency that's covered by insurance, or other help that might be needed in the home. Make sure you understand **everything** that you'll need, and how to get it ordered and delivered quickly, before you and your charge get back home.

You may also need to get specific medical equipment for continuing care, such as a cane, walker, lift/stand recliner, gait belt, wheelchair, hospital bed, air mattress, medical lift, portable commode, or other equipment. Make a list of what's needed immediately. Hospital discharge personnel will likely be able to assist or direct you to where you can rent or purchase necessary equipment.

Small items that are not critical to day-to-day well-being can be ordered and purchased online and can typically mean a wait of only a few days.

For non-essential, but "good to have" items (e.g., stand-lift lounge chairs and footstool, etc.), take the time to shop around for where you can purchase or rent necessary equipment. Equipment costs can vary widely, and used equipment, in good shape, may work just fine.

Note: *Equipment costs can add up quickly. Check with your insurance company to assess what equipment costs are covered. If your charge is not fully insurance-covered and a veteran, you may be able to get much of it covered through the Veterans Administration. However, firm, persistent follow-through and monitoring of the progress of your request with VA personnel may be required to keep things from falling through the cracks.*

If you know friends, relatives, or neighbors whose family members used but no longer need such equipment, ask if you can borrow or buy what they may still have around and no longer need.

Check your local Goodwill, Salvation Army, and other gently used item stores in your area for non-essential equipment. You'll likely be surprised as to what you can find there. Being resourceful at this stage of need may serve you, and your charge, well.

Discharged to a Care Facility

The hospital may recommend that you transfer your charge to one of several types of care facilities. The type of facility will depend on the outcomes from the emergency and the prognosis of your charge's health condition and situation.

Skilled Nursing and Rehabilitation Care Facilities

These types of facilities typically provide services that focus on temporary rehabilitation that does not require long-term care, including physical therapy, occupational therapy, and speech therapy. Depending on their license, these facilities often have licensed medical professionals on site, 24/7. A skilled nursing or rehabilitation facility is typically recommended to help your charge learn how to manage on their own (or with the right support) outside of a hospital setting. You may, however, be able get physical therapy, occupational therapy, and/or speech therapy provided in your charge's home, too.

If, after the emergency or hospital stay, medical personnel recommend your charge be released to one of these facilities, you may want to consider being there or having an aide, family member, or some assistants with them 24/7 for a few days. Doing so may give you time to assess the facility and make sure it is the right place for your charge. Having someone with them 24/7 will also help you better understand how much their condition has changed and what type of accommodations you may have to make at home or where you will need to bring them next. This may be an assisted living, memory care, or skilled nursing facility.

Although having 24/7 oversight in a rehabilitation or other type of facility may give you some peace of mind, accidents can happen when least expected, even in a facility you think is fully monitored and safe. **Hospital, or an incident-induced delirium**, can

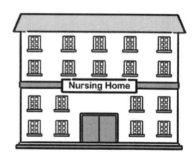

set in and result in fear, anxiety, depression, or confusion and **cause unexpected reactions from your charge**. Many unintentional situations can occur such as falls, bed sores, and hygiene issues. This may be due to many causes, including inadequate staff support. If you are uncertain of the care they're getting, we recommend **having someone at their side** to reduce potential life-threatening problems, anxiety, or fear, until both you and your charge are comfortable with their care.

Discharged to a Custodial Care Facility

Nursing homes and **assisted living facilities** provide long-term custodial care assistance, typically simple medical, but mostly non-medical, care. This includes support with basic day-to-day needs like general hygiene care (bathing and bathroom assistance), meals, housekeeping needs, some medication management, general safety monitoring, transportation to and from medical appointments, and some entertainment available to residents. These facilities, based on their license, may have medical professionals on site full or part time.

You may be asked to make a quick decision on which facility to send your charge to, without knowing much about them, including the quality of care they provide.

Most hospitals will work to recommend a reputable local nursing or assisted care facility, but it is ultimately your responsibility to make sure it is the right place for your charge. Do your own independent reputational check, too.

Speak with the facility administration before arranging transportation, and review all documentation. Take time to fully understand your financial obligations, insurance coverage, and rights with the facility. Get details about the exact type of care your charge will be receiving and if that meets the hospital discharge recommendations.

It's just as important to know what type of notice you have to give to move your charge to a new facility if the one you've selected does not work out. This includes notice they are required to give you, should they decide that they are not able to properly care for your charge.

As with any legal document, take time to thoroughly read and understand all papers that you will be signing before your charge is transported to the facility. If you do not understand even the simplest points of the intake documents that you've been given, ask. **This is not a time to be shy about getting more details or explanations on what you don't fully comprehend**.

Once your charge has been transferred to the facility (as noted in the section on skilled nursing and rehabilitation facilities), if you can, spend several days monitoring their transition. This will give you an opportunity to request changes to the type and amount of care they may need to keep them mentally, emotionally, and physically comfortable and safe. Knowing they will be well cared for, when you are not at their side, should provide you with greater peace of mind and comfort, too.

Memory Care Facilities

Many continued care facilities, which typically include independent and assisted living living options, also have a memory care unit, wing or floor. There are also those facilities that specialize in the needs of those who have dementia and Alzheimer's or other severe cognitive issues that make it difficult for them to live at home or in a facility with less support or care.

Not all memory care facilities are the same in the types and qualities of care offered. However, they should all have locked or alarmed doors to prevent your charge from wandering outside the facility unattended, ways to monitor falls, support with meals and eating (when needed), as well as all the additional care services offered by an assisted care facility. This includes help with the daily chores of life: dressing, bathing, toileting, eating, transferring, mobility, housekeeping, medication management, transportation to/from medical appointments (or an in-house medical team), and social engagement, at the very least.

Discharged to Hospice

Hospice services are meant to make the end-of-life process easier for your charge. If you and your doctor have agreed that placing your charge in hospice care is the next step, then there are some options from which you can choose: hospice at home or in the facility where they presently reside, or in a separate facility run and managed by a hospice.

Depending on the area where your charge lives, you may have a choice of hospice providers. However, many smaller communities only have one hospice care provider servicing the area.

The hospice provider can be a not-for-profit or for-profit organization. Many hospitals have a hospice representative at their facility to help you understand the whole process, the documents that you'll need to sign, what's covered by insurance, and what liabilities you or your charge may have when agreeing to hospice care. In addition, they will help you decide on the option of transferring your charge to a hospice managed facility or taking them home. They will also give you and your family and/or caregivers instructions on how to provide the most comfort and care to your charge.

Hospice at home may be easier for your charge. However, it may be emotionally and physically draining on everyone around them. You should take time to fully understand what to expect, and how much you will have to do to properly care for your charge at home. You will also need a solid support team that can give you time out to sleep, eat, and care for yourself. A good hospice agency will help you understand just how much you can manage yourself and if/when you need additional help.

At this point, it's important to understand that you are working to manage the comfort of your charge in their final months, weeks, days, and hours. This includes helping them with bathing, toileting (if possible) and incontinence issues, constipation (you may have to give them a suppository), wound management, respiratory care, pain management/medication, and nutritional and hydration needs. All of the above will be more complex for you, the caregiver, in helping your charge get through their final time with dignity and grace.

Before you agree to a hospice facility, make sure it is Medicare certified. You may also want to research the ratings and reviews by families who have used the hospice's services in the past. Don't just look at the worst and best ratings. The middle ratings may give you a more realistic or balanced perspective on what to expect.

Call and talk to the hospice managers so that you are comfortable with what they say they will provide. This is your time to also voice any concerns, discuss complaints that you may have read online, and get a better understanding of what might have transpired.

In general, families who have worked with hospices are thankful for their care and support in the final stages of life.

Hospice facility or hospice "house": These facilities are typically designed to provide a home-like environment for your charge. They may only be available for a short time, but do offer you the comfort of knowing that 24/7 skilled care is on-site for your charge.

If you are limited in the time for which your charge can stay at a hospice facility, and they survive beyond that time, then you will likely be required to take them home. At that point, you will be the one managing care, with the support of local hospice care management teams.

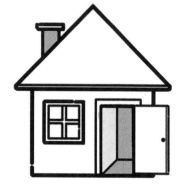

Some people spend time in, out, and back in hospice facilities. This is emotionally and physically challenging. Being prepared for this type of in-out-in again is something you may want to plan for, based on what is offered and available through the hospice facility in your area.

While there is much more that we could cover on how to select and assess facilities, the points covered in this section should give you some guidance to get your charge transferred from the hospital to the type of facility the hospital recommends in support of their specific type of care needs.

There are other services available to you, the caregiver and your charge, through hospice. This includes a non-denominational spiritual advisor and/or chaplain and social worker. You should always be able to reach a medical professional (nurse, physician's assistant, or doctor) 24/7 via phone. The ability for someone to physically visit your charge may be limited based on the number of patients they have assigned to each hospice team member, the needs of the other patient or families, the time of day, the day of the week (weekends may have different or fewer staff members), or level of care urgency.

The hospice process can be physically and emotionally draining to the caregiver and family. As difficult as it may be, take time to step away occasionally, catch your breath, and get out (e.g., get some sun, take a walk, etc.). Even though it may seem difficult, taking short breaks may make the final moments with your charge a bit easier.

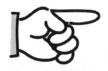

What's Next For Your Charge Summary

- Consider the discharge process as a new starting point for you and your charge. Understand why the emergency occurred and how to move on or into a new phase of care.

- Your charge (and you, with POA) can discharge yourself anytime you wish. But the hospital will likely not accept any possible risk for doing so.

- You may be able to speed up discharge if you understand the process, such as: finding out who's in charge, asking for progress reports, and helping to do tasks like retrieving printouts from the printer.

- Get a print out of all discharge papers. Read carefully. Get explanations. Don't sign what you do not agree with.

- Try to anticipate where the hospital will recommend sending your charge, so that you start to arrange transport as necessary.

- If discharged home, make arrangements to adapt the home to any new caring needs.

- If discharged to a temporary care facility, check the facility out and have someone stay with your charge to understand if it's the right, and safe, place to be.

- If discharged to a custodial facility, keep regular monitoring on your charge's health and treatment.

- If discharged to hospice, determine if home hospice is more appropriate than in a facility.

What's Next for You?

Going through a medical emergency can be difficult for your charge, but it can also be stressful and difficult for your charge's family, friends, and, even more so, you, their caregiver. It's important to reflect on why the emergency happened, what missteps — if any — were made, and where preparations could have been better. From that reflection, one can gain knowledge to improve one's caregiving.

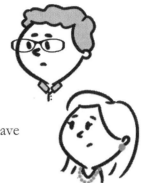

It's also important to assess what effects going through the emergency with your charge may have had (and may still be having) on you. This is an important, but often neglected, aspect of caregiving: family caregivers taking care of themselves.

The following are some suggestions and ways for you to start to "recover" from the experience and stress of caring for your charge during their medical emergency.

Learning From the Experience
No two 911 emergency situations are exactly the same. If you've followed the points in this book, you used your journal/notebook to summarize everything that happened along the way. While fresh in your mind, add to your notes by listing what went well, where you got frustrated or hit roadblocks, what didn't go well, and how you might be better prepared for the next time.

Updating Your Skills
Get training or help on how to better manage those areas where you were unsure of what to do. If you managed the situation but thought you could have done better, review with others or research the ways others have done similar things. One example is to practice "what if" scenarios with those you trust, similar to those fire drills

we participated in at school or at work. Practicing and refreshing your skills before the next emergency will increase your confidence so that you can help your charge and others when the next time comes.

Getting More Support

The stress from a medical emergency can also take its toll on you physically and psychologically, and on those around you. Recovering from it may take more time than you think.

Join a support group, talk with family members, or get help from religious advisors, social workers, or someone else you trust who is familiar with caregiver and family life stress. Being able to confidentially speak about what you've gone through and getting other perspectives on how to cope may be just what you need.

Focus on Getting Yourself Back Together

As the old saying goes, "We must be able to care for ourselves, before we can care for others." Don't think of this as selfish, but as sensible. If you, as a caregiver, are hurting or ill, your ability to help your charge suffers.

Take time to fully assess the impact the emergency has had on you:

Physically, have you:

- ❏ Lost or gained weight?
- ❏ Been eating lots of food that are bad for you?
- ❏ Seen a shift in mood swings?
- ❏ Not been able to sleep or get enough sleep?
- ❏ Neglected your own health warning signs?

Emotionally, have you:

- ❏ Avoided friends and family?
- ❏ Snapped at someone more than once in the past day?

- ☐ Started back on old bad habits like smoking?
- ☐ Increased a habit to try and eliminate the pain of stress?
- ☐ Lost trust in those around you?
- ☐ Micromanaged more than usual?
- ☐ Gone shopping just to buy things you don't need, hoping that it might make you feel better?

Financially, have you:

- ☐ Had to take unpaid time off from work?
- ☐ Postponed client work (if an entrepreneur)?
- ☐ Neglected bills?

Spiritually, have you:

- ☐ Not spent time with the community that makes you feel good about yourself?
- ☐ Not asked for guidance when most needed?
- ☐ Not had, nor spent enough quiet time to allow your mind and heart to relax (even a bit) and try to heal?

The Good and Bad of Self-Soothing

We all like to feel good. Self-soothing is natural and important to healing. Treating ourselves and our loved ones to a special experience or day out can work wonders for both of you. However, falling into traps and habits to feel temporarily better can become emotionally, physically, and financially debilitating.

Keep note on what makes you feel good and why. If it's a simple pleasure that cannot cause long-term harm, go at it! If it's something that can cause you physical or psychological harm over time, get outside help to support you over the stressful time so that you're able to find joy on your own in different ways.

Working to Get Whole Again

Working to "get whole again" varies for everyone. For you, this may mean a walk in the park with your dog, spending quiet time on the couch with a pet, and so forth. Note: Pets are a recognized way to help lower your blood pressure and calm your nerves. However, keeping a pet is a long term responsibility and commitment. Don't get one just to help yourself feel better and recover.

Try taking the time to get a massage, manicure, or facial. Learn to meditate. Practice box breathing to slow you down and relax your nerves **(https://www.medicalnewstoday.com/articles/321805)**.

Hard physical and aerobic exercise (if you're physically capable) is another way that has been scientifically proven to reduce stress, anxiety, and restlessness. Try it!

Get fresh air and sunshine for at least 30 minutes a day. If easy to achieve, take your charge with you for a walk, or if they're incapable of walking, push their wheelchair around the block, or for a stroll around the mall.

These are just a few examples of how you can start to reclaim your head, heart, and energy again.

Build Your Social Network

We are social creatures, and isolation can harm us in more ways than we think. Building a diverse network of creative, intelligent, fun, and supportive people will make the time you spend as a caregiver more rich and enjoyable. A diverse social network will also help you become a more creative problem solver, as, in all likelihood, some of those in your network have experienced caring for a loved one at some point too.

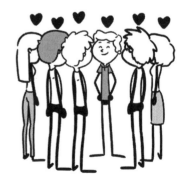

Share your feelings and experience and ask for ideas on how best to address what you're managing. You might be surprised where and when your best solutions present themselves. Invite some or all of your social network for lunch or dinner, together with your charge. Make it an event that they, and your charge, will likely laugh and smile about for a long time to come.

Reflection

Take time to think about all the good that you've done to help your charge through the 911 emergency. Share how excited you are with all the good that resulted with your charge. Bring them into the process so that, together, you're better, happier, and more efficient (when possible) day in and day out.

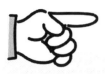

What's Next For You Summary

- Review all notes you took during the emergency.

- Assess what went well, what didn't, and what things you need to get fixed or learn to better prepare for the future.

- Update and expand your skills where needed.

- Discuss the emergency with others and how you can, together, improve your caregiving.

- Do a self-assessment. Be extra vigilant of changes that have happened, changes to your habits and routines, and how you feel physically and mentally since the emergency.

- Avoid destructive self-soothing: habits that cause weight gain or damage your health usually start out as feeling good. Make a list of the things that make you feel good and compare them against those that are good for you.

- Seek help and support from those you trust or from those professionals who you think can help you.

- Build or rebuild your social network. Work to expand mutual help networks for the future.

- Reflect on the good things that you were able to do for your charge in the emergency. A well-deserved pat on the back, even only from yourself, is still a good thing.

5

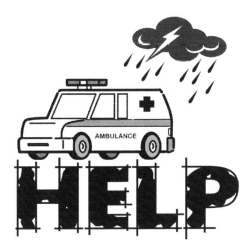

Getting Help in a Time of Disaster

Save the Lives of Life Savers

Recent events have proved that our first responders and medical professionals are critical to getting life-saving care to us when we need it. Unfortunately, since they often place themselves in danger doing so, they get injured, exposed to infections, and even die from trying to help us. It is important that we always remember that their safety is critical, too.

In any emergency situation, if you or your charge, is or has been exposed to any infectious or life-threatening disease, or you know that there are conditions where first responders could be injured or sickened, it is critical to alert the dispatcher and hospital administrators so that responders and medical personnel can be equipped with the proper tools and their own personal safety protection before providing care.

Getting Help During Disasters

In the previous chapters, we highlighted actions and plans to get you through an emergency better in normal times. However, things change when a disaster hits. To paraphrase a famous quote: t*he best laid plans often go astray*. Disasters can be game changers for those needing immediate emergency medical care. In the US alone, the Federal Emergency Management Agency (FEMA), has responded to an average of 130 disasters per year over the last 10 years.

Disasters can take many forms and be widespread, as with hurricanes, tornados, snowstorms, earthquakes, mass shootings, system-wide power failures, pandemics, etc. They can also be localized, down to a city, town, several blocks or single buildings. Even if the event affects only a few, it can still be a disaster for those going through it.

In such cases, your local hospital, healthcare facilities, or even regional healthcare systems may be overwhelmed. This could also happen with first responders, disaster crews, and infrastructure such as power, telecommunications, and roadways — all of which we depend on. Although many hospital emergency departments can scale up quickly, they may be unprepared at first for a catastrophe. Even worse, hospitals themselves could be devastated by a disaster such as when Hurricane Katrina flooded hospitals in Louisiana.

Unfortunately, because there may be so many variables, it could be very difficult to plan for everything that could go wrong. Even with the best professional scenario planning, unforeseen things can get in the way of getting help to you and your charge, quickly.

You can pretty much divide all disasters into two groups: those where you would be better off evacuating to a shelter or facility, and those where you would shelter and stay in your home. In cases where you would get some advance notice before a disaster hit — like a hurricane, flood, or approaching fire, civil unrest etc., you may have time to evacuate or be moved to a safer location. In instances where there is no notice, like an earthquake, tornado, or sudden severe weather, you may have no choice, or it might be better, as in a pandemic, to stay in your home. If you have frail, infirm, or special needs charges, the decision to evacuate to where help is readily available should, in most cases be the wiser choice. Of course, you need to put together an evacuation kit to ensure that your charge has what they need to sustain them. You can find sample tips at **https://www.fema.gov/media-library/assets/documents/90354**.

In this chapter, we highlight some disaster-related challenges that could arise for family caregivers, who are sheltering in their or somebody's home during a disaster and whose charges subsequently need immediate medical attention. These situations may raise more challenges in getting medical help than what has been discussed in the previous chapters. We've laid out additional suggestions obtained from first responders on how to work through such challenges. It's also important to note that the tools and actions previously mentioned in this book (File of Life, Go Bag, First Aid Kit, support networks, etc.), are just as important to have, use, and follow in getting you and your charge through a disaster better.

Communicating in a Disaster

Reaching Help in a Disaster When 911 Seems To Be Down

During a disaster, the 911 system could go down in your area or be totally overwhelmed. However, you may still be able make cell and landline calls. When there is a 911 outage in your area, you may receive an alerting call informing you of your local or regional emergency responders' non-emergency numbers. If you get such a call, immediately check that you have already posted them or write them down and put them up in a conspicuous place.

Try This:

- ❑ If you know or believe 911 is down, don't keep trying to call 911. Instead, call your local non-emergency fire or police department numbers, and follow the process outlined in **Chapter 3** for making a 911 call.

- ❑ If you don't have or know the non-emergency numbers, call the "information" number on your cell or landline phone. This process may delay you getting help, but you will still be doing something to get help.

- ❑ If possible, get others in the household, or even a neighbor to make this call, while you focus on helping your charge.

Plan Before It Happens:

- ❑ Write down non-emergency fire and police phone numbers near or right at the top of your File of Life and post them where you can see them easily, like on the refrigerator.

- ❑ Add these numbers into your cell phone contacts list.

- ☐ Do this right now, before reading further.

Reaching Help in a Disaster When Cell Phone Service Is Not Working

In a disaster cell phone service may become unreliable, spotty, or stop altogether. Always check your signal strength before using your phone. Other phone services such as landlines (copper wired is typically the most reliable), cable or VOIP can also become compromised. However, these systems may have better backup power than the cell phone service in your area.

Try This:

- ☐ Quickly, check that you have a cell phone signal or your phone is actually charged or working.

- ☐ If you have no cell service, try to get to the nearest landline phone and call 911.

- ☐ See if anyone else immediately close by can make a cell phone call or landline emergency call for you.

- ☐ Even if cell service is out, you can try using Text-to-911. Text-to-911 is a FCC-managed service that allows text messages to go through to a central emergency call center, even if cell service is not operating. This program is available in most but not all communities, in the US.

- ☐ If nothing else works, try to get your charge by yourself, or with the help of others, to a place where you can be seen and get help, or all the way to a hospital.

Plan Before It Happens:

- ☐ If affordable, consider installing or reactivating landline service installed in the house, even if just as a backup.

- ☐ Make sure the handset you want to use does not require electrical plug-in power.

- ☐ Confirm whether you have text-to-911 service available in your area.

❑ Post a Text-to-911 reminder next to your File of Life, on the front of side of your refrigerator.

Note: *A list of communities that offer this service can be found at:* **https://www.fcc.gov/file/12285/download**. *If your community is NOT listed, check with your local police and responders, as the list is updated monthly.*

❑ If your charge doesn't have landline phone service in their home, ask around and make note of who has landline service near you.

❑ Get to know which of your neighbors may be willing to help out in an emergency. It is unlikely they will refuse to let you make a call in an emergency.

Getting and Giving Help in a Disaster When I Can't Move My Charge and I Can't Reach Anyone to Help Me

In some cases, where no one is close by and all forms of communication are out, you may not be able to reach help at all.

Try This:

❑ When you can, run or go to a neighbor for help. If you live close to a neighboring house, or are in an apartment or condo complex, go to your neighbors for assistance.

❑ Don't give up. Go outside when you can and loudly yell for help. Wave a cloth, shine a flashlight, or do whatever you can to flag help down.

❑ If you can't move or leave your charge alone, make and place a large white sheet or board with the words HELP, or NEED DOCTOR on it in VERY LARGE AND BOLD LETTERS, where it can easily be seen. This may be outside the front door of a house or hung from a street-facing window.

Plan Before It Happens:

- Get to know your neighbors and which ones you can rely on to help in a disaster emergency

- Create an informal emergency network group. Make sure that everyone in your group agrees to a plan and process for checking on one another throughout a disaster period.

- Keep at least one white sheet or large cloth along with a VERY large permanent marker in your First Aid kit.

- Make sure the words written on the sheet could be easily seen from a long distance (foot-high letters are only readable up to 500 feet away).

- In preparation for an impending disaster, you may want to create this type of flag/signal well in advance, so that it's ready for use, if needed.

Reaching Help in a Disaster When Electrical Power is Out

In a disaster, the electric service to your home or area may not work. This could be due to a disaster-caused power failure, downed wires, or have been deliberately cut off by the power company itself. However, cell phones and landline phones may still work.

Try This:

- Check to see if your cell phone still works. Call 911. Also advise the dispatcher if you see power lines down outside.

- Make sure to turn off all apps that use power so you don't run out your battery quickly.

- If your cell phone is out and you DO have a landline phone, check to see that it is working. Call 911.

- Check the neighborhood to see who has power and/or phone service, and can help, or get you help.

Note: *Some landlines need an electrical plug for a power source. If that's the case, make sure you have a remote battery backup that you can plug the phone into. If your phone does not need to be plugged into an electric outlet, you may be able to call 911 or others for help even with no electric power.*

Plan Before It Happens:

- ☐ If you have landline service, get an old-fashioned simple phone that doesn't need power — like a princess phone.

- ☐ Get and keep several remote battery backup devices for charging your cell phones in a pinch. Make sure they are always fully charged.

- ☐ Get an extra cell phone car-charger, or a USB car-charger connection cord as a backup phone charging option.

Getting Help in a Disaster When Electrical Power is Out, and You Use Life-Sustaining Equipment

If your charge relies on powered life-sustaining equipment, it's wise to always have some form of backup power, alternative non-powered equipment, or a plan to get your charge to a location that has access to power. Note: in some locations you may have to share a power source with other critical-needs individuals in extreme situations.

If you've registered with your local utility's Emergency Medical Equipment Notification Program and registered with local first responders, don't count on their being able to restore power to you timely or make you a priority for power restoration. In addition, do not expect that they or others can deliver any form of backup power equipment to you, when you need it.

Try This:

- ☐ Check to see if the power outage is widespread.

- ☐ If you can move your charge, check to see if you, a neighbor, or the building you live in, has a working generator that is safe to hook your charges life-sustaining equipment up to.

- ☐ If you can reach the utility company, and/or first responders, call and let them know you're in a critical care/life-sustaining equipment emergency situation.

- ☐ If nothing else works, and it's feasible to move your charge, you may need to try getting them, by yourself or with the help of others, to a place where you can get power, be seen and get help, or if necessary all the way to a powered facility.

Plan Before It Happens:

- ☐ Register your charge with your local utility's *Emergency Medical Equipment Notification Program* and first responders as a person needing assistance in a disaster situation.

- ☐ Talk with your healthcare providers about alternatives to using power-reliant life-sustaining medical equipment and what else can be done to keep your charge alive in the event of a power failure.

- ☐ Ensure that your charge has some type of medical ID indicating the need for specific life-sustaining equipment and/or medications.

- ☐ If you choose to have an electric generator/inverter or other remote power source in your home, make **absolutely sure** you completely understand how to safely operate and attach medical equipment to it.

   Note: *Generators and inverters require regular maintenance, testing, and sources of fuel. This could be propane, gasoline, diesel, or solar power. These fuel sources also need to be checked and maintained. These devices should NEVER BE OPERATED INDOORS AND SHOULD ALWAYS BE PROPERLY GROUNDED.*

Getting and Giving Help in a Disaster When Responders May Not be Able to Get to Me

Sometimes, responders cannot physically get to you right away, due to downed trees, wires, floods, etc. If an ambulance cannot physically get to your location, a larger, heavier fire truck or equipment may be able to reach you. If a fire truck can't get through, they may try to use other means like an ATV, helicopter, road-clearing equipment, or even walking in with a crew and stretcher. In most cases EMTs, firefighters, and police will do nearly anything they can to get to you, providing it does not put their life in absolute peril. These people have an innate drive to run into danger, but they also know their limits in being able to get to you and get you to a hospital safely. In such situations, patience, and some self-reliance can go a long way in getting you help more quickly.

Try This:

- ❏ If you've reached a dispatcher, answered all their questions, and followed their directions, and you believe it may be a while before a responder can physically get to you, make sure to get the dispatcher's name before you hang up the phone. This may save you time (by not having to repeat all the information you've already shared), if you need to call back and to relay changes in your charge's condition or need to get updates on responders progress in getting to you.

- ❏ If your charge can be temporarily left alone, or someone else in the home can assist, safely try and assess what conditions are outside that could potentially obstruct or prevent responders from getting to you and your charge.

- ❏ If you or someone else can help to clear obstructions, do so only if **you know what you're doing and you are absolutely sure that you can do so safely.**

- ❏ **Do not assume that downed wires are unpowered!**

Plan Before It Happens:

- ❑ As an addendum to your home walkthrough, mentioned in **Chapter 1**, observe and try to envision what on or around the home property, street, and neighborhood, could potentially become obstructions to responders in a disaster.

- ❑ Keep heavy work gloves and safety glasses in or near your First Aid kit.

- ❑ Purchase and keep a battery powered radio or TV and spare batteries. Ocassionally test to make sure they will work properly when needed.

- ❑ Keep extra small device batteries, and a few bottles of water available at all times.

Getting Help In A Disaster When You've Been Told There Are No Ambulances Available

The emergency crews in your area may become overwhelmed with other calls, if your responders are overwhelmed with calls: Emergency responder crews and departments are all closely aligned and connected to other crews in the regional area. If your local responders are flooded with calls they will find a way to get someone to you from a supporting town, or from another responder group in your community to come to your aid.

If an ambulance cannot get to you right away, your local responder team will do what they can to reach you. If your town or community is overwhelmed, they will work to find the next available and closest responder to help you. However, if in your case, the emergency responders are overwhelmed, and they can't receive additional help from a nearby town or emergency crew, you may have to wait. In this case, it's critical to tell the dispatcher the details and extent of your urgency. An immediate

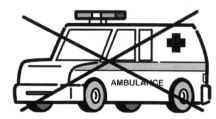

life-threatening situation will likely get moved up in the response queue, over one that is not life-threatening, but there is no guarantee. Typically 911 responses are on a first-come-first-serve, unless they otherwise tell you something different.

Try This:

- ❏ Make sure the dispatcher knows exactly what is going on with your charge. Understand that what may seem like an emergency to you, may be less so to them based on what emergency calls they are receiving.

- ❏ Listen to what the dispatcher is telling you. DO NOT hang up until you're told to do so!

- ❏ Ask for an estimated time of arrival (ETA) for responders if they can provide one.

Plan Before It Happens:

- ❏ It's absolutely important that you keep up or even advance your first aid and CPR skills. This is especially true if you are the only person available to provide life-saving support to your charge, while waiting for responders to arrive.

- ❏ It's helpful to know which responder facilities are closest to you and your charge's home so that you can let a dispatcher know, especially if they do not know the area.

Getting Help In A Disaster When the Hospital Is Closed or Has Reached Over Capacity

Most, if not all hospitals, have a maximum capacity of patients they can serve at any one time, even in a disaster. If, in a disaster, they are not able to set up additional ways to support patient demand, they will likely direct those in need to other facilities (even temporary triage facilities and tents). Hospitals are the epicenter in many disaster scenarios, and have plans in place to direct patients to other facilities. If this happens, get the name, location, and address of where your charge will be transported before the ambulance leaves your home with them. Give your phone number to the transporting driver, in case they are redirected to an alternate facility. You do not want to lose track of where your charge is in a disaster.

Try This:

- ❏ **Always keep your charge's File of Life with them.** Ensure it is securely attached to their clothing whenever they leave with an emergency response team.

- ❏ It may also be helpful to write, in permanent marker, their name, date of birth, and your contact phone number on their arm, leg or clothing, so that someone can contact you, should their File of Life get lost or misplaced.

- ❏ Check your cell phone for GPS service to see if you can locate exactly where responders intend to take your charge.

- ❏ If you don't have a GPS service, try to find a printed map of your area that identifies where responders said they will be taking your charge.

Plan Before It Happens:

- ☐ Make sure you have up-to-date Files of Life.

- ☐ Keep a permanent marker in your Go Bag and First Aid kit at all times.

- ☐ Keep a local printed map in your Go Bag with hospital locations in your area circled on the map.

- ☐ Make sure you have all these hospital phone numbers in your cell phone contacts, and written right on the map.

Staying in Contact When You're not Allowed to Stay With Your Charge Once at The Hospital

In many disaster situations, hospitals will not allow non-patient individuals to enter the building, beyond the admissions area. This can become especially problematic for those who have charges with dementia or other form of cognitive challenges. Unfortunately, there may be little you can do to resolve this issue yourself. Some hospitals in disaster situations may have in-house Certified Nursing Assistants (CNA) or technicians who can help keep your charge at ease.

Try This:

- ☐ Try to get the direct dial phone number for the emergency department desk.
- ☐ Give them your phone number so they can contact you for critical medical decisions.
- ☐ Tell the responders and admitting medical personnel about your charge's cognitive and emotional state.
- ☐ Make sure a File of Life is securely attached to their clothing or tucked into a pocket.
- ☐ Find out from the hospital what the process is for keeping in contact with your charge or how they will keep you informed about their medical status.
- ☐ If your charge is capable of using a cell phone, make sure they have one with them, along with a power supply charger.

Plan Before It Happens:

- ☐ Make sure you always have an up-to-date File of Life that you can send with your charge.
- ☐ Keep a permanent pen or marker in your Go Bag so you can quickly print pertinent information on your charge's arm, leg or clothing, if necessary.

- ☐ Find out what the communication policies and procedures are for your local medical facilities.

- ☐ Get an inexpensive prepaid cell phone and charger that you can give to your charge. In many cases hospital security may not allow them to keep such devices with them or they may simply get lost or stolen.

Final Note

Medical 911 emergencies can take a huge toll on you, the caregiver, your family, and support team. They are **never easy** and, rarely, if ever, the same the next time around.

Being prepared for what to expect, what to do, and how to respond, may help reduce your stress in any given emergency situation. Your preparation and ability to manage stress will better help your charge through the experience and recovery process.

Being prepared for a 911 medical emergency, and knowing how to support responders and the emergency department medical team, is even more critical when disasters strike. Those who are prepared and know what to do, how to get help, and are emotionally and physically prepared will be in a far better positoin to help their charges than someone who's not.

Even if you manage to only put a few of the suggestions in this guide into practice, you will be more capable of helping responders and medical teams get you and your charge through an emergency more successfully.

Be well, be safe, be prepared.

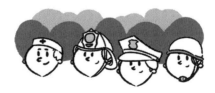

Special Thanks

Special thanks has to go out to all those who contributed their ideas, thoughts, critiques, and content, format, and editorial suggestions to develop this guide book: Bonnie Annis; Alexandra Chalif, MS, MP; extra appreciation to Bruce Jones, Elizabeth Stuart Fullerton, Adele Hanks RN, Gerit Quealey, Roxanne Khazarian, John Iannuzzi, Mildred Martinez (love you lots), every single one of the very special Fab 5 women, Sarah Senkus RN, Dmitrii Pisarenko, Sally Baker, Heather Gaynor, Matthew Forbes Erskine, Esq., Nathaniel Erskine, MD, the EMT instructor and quiet friend, Bruce Y. Lee, MD, George Antonion, Cpt. D. J. Skelton, US Army (Retired), Ellen Goodwin, Joan Mohin, PhD, Natalie Silver, Lynn Maria Thompson, Samantha Nichols, Alex Nichols, Assistant Fire Chief, family members, friends, and so many more.

About the Authors

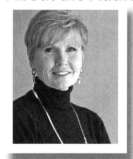

Nancy May

Nancy May has spent her career working with CEOs, Boards of Directors, and senior leaders in the public and private sectors. These experiences gave her the strength and foundation to step in and provide her parents with guidance and support, both as their POA and Trustee, as they aged. She credits her father, an entrepreneur and innovator in eyewear design, and her mom, for encouraging and preparing her to acquire the many skills needed to start and lead several successful businesses. She has transitioned these competencies and life lessons to into her new business, CareManity, LLC, which focuses on providing family caregivers structured ways to obtain practical knowledge and access much-needed support.

Robert W. Antonion

Robert Antonion has been a first responder, management auditor, corporate governance researcher and analyst, and business writer. As a responder, he received numerous awards and recognitions for his work. As a supporting member of CareManity, LLC, he prefers to provide, in the background, detailed research, added dimension, and even emotional strength and a level of sanity to others in the company during hectic times He's also camera shy.

READER NOTES

Your Go Bag

Made in the USA
Columbia, SC
12 March 2023